Gut Balance Revolution & Blood Pressure Solution
Omnibus

By

Dermot Farrell

www.healbodymindandspirit.com

Foreword to Gut Balance Revolution & Blood Pressure Solution Omnibus

In this omnibus you are getting two books in one.

The first book Gut Health covers a wide range of herbs which can treat the following conditions:

- Leaky Gut Syndrome
- Heartburn
- Diarrhoea
- Constipation
- Peptic ulcers
- Stomach sensitivity
- Irritable Bowel Syndrome (IBS)

And in the second book Blood Pressure Solution it covers natural approaches towards regulating your blood pressure levels, which includes such strategies as:

- Lifestyle changes
- Traditional Chinese Medical cures
- Pranayama (Yogic breathing techniques)
- Herbal cures
- Hatha yoga Asana's

Between these two books, there is a huge amount of information which is all backed up with academic research and footnotes, so you know you're not getting waffle!

Regular allopathic medicine has its place in health care, but before the modern pharmaceutical revolution took off our grandparents and great grand parents did a good job of treating their health conditions naturally. So why rely solely upon drugs when you can use natural herbal remedies, Chinese medicine, hatha yoga and pranayama and positive life changes to treat your health!

Finally not only will natural treatments help your health problems, but also because they are tonic like in nature, they boost health and vitality levels thus helping you not only to treat chronic health issues but also to become a healthier and happier individual in the process and of course herbs are pretty cheap and easily accessible.

Contents

Foreword to Gut Balance Revolution & Blood Pressure Solution Omnibus	1
Book 1 - Gut Balance Revolution	8
Free Gifts	11
Introduction	12
Chapter One – Why is your Gut in Such a Mess!!!	14
Some Common Stomach/Gut Health Conditions Causes	17
Chapter Two – Good Habits for Everyone to Follow	21
Simple Food Advice	21
General Good Eating Habits	26
Chapter Three – Common Gut Health Problems and How to Treat Them	32
Foods which are good for Gut Health	32
Supplements for Gut Health	45
Chapter Four - Gut Healing Program	59

Chart One	60
Chart Two	63
Detox	64
Final Thoughts on Gut Health Rebalancing	74
Appendix – 28 Day Gut Restoration Program	76
Food preliminaries	77
Three meals a Day	79
Detox Shakes and Juices	80
Micronutrient Meal	80
Macronutrient Meal	80
Supplementation	97
Summing up the 28 Day Gut Restoration Program	98
Thank You	102
BOOK 2 - BLOOD PRESSURE SOLUTION	103
Medical Disclaimer	104
PART ONE – OVERVIEW	106
CHAPTER ONE – GETTING A HANDLE ON YOUR HIGH BLOOD PRESSURE	
	107

CHAPTER TWO - HIGH BLOOD PRESSURE POTENTIAL DANGERS AND CAUSES

117

ALLOPATHIC CAUSES 120

TRADITIONAL CHINESE MEDICINE CAUSES 122

A WORD OF WARNING! 128

WHERE ALLOPATHY MEETS TCM 129

PART TWO – PRACTICAL STRATEGIES 132

CHAPTER THREE - LIFESTYLE CHANGES 133

PALEO DIET/HIGH FAT/LOW CARB/KETOGENIC DIETS – CHOLESTEROL IS GOOD FOR YOU ETC.????? 141

THE IMPORTANCE OF EXERCISE AND GENERAL LIFESTYLE CHANGES 147

HOW TO FIND HAPPINESS IN A CRAZY WORLD 154

SUMMING UP LIFESTYLE CHANGES 169

CHAPTER FOUR – PRANAYAMA 173

BASIC RULES AND CONTRAINDICATIONS 174

A SERIOUS WARNING!!! 175

MEDICAL RESEARCH CONFIRMS THE EFFECTIVENESS OF PRANAYAMA'S

178

CHAPTER FIVE - HATHA YOGA 190

SAVASANNA 190

PASCHIMOTTANASANA (FORWARD BEND POSE) 191

SHASHANKASANA (HARE POSE) AND BALASANA POSE (POSE OF A CHILD) 193

TRADITIONAL CHINESE POISES	198
THE CRANE, THE TURTLE AND THE SOLAR PLEXUS EXERCISES	199
CHAPTER SIX - HERBAL CURES	208
WALNUTS AND HONEY	209
CINNAMON	209
GARLIC	211
GINGER	213
CARDAMOM	216
RAUVOLFIA SERPENTINA	218
CONCLUSION – PUTTING IT ALL TOGETHER	221
FREE GIFTS	228
Thank You	228
APPENDIX	230

Gut Balance Solution

By

Dermot Farrell

www.healbodymindandspirit.com

Copyright © 2017 and beyond Dermot Farrell

All Rights Reserved. No part of this publication may be reproduced in any form or by any means, including scanning, photocopying, or otherwise without prior written permission of the copyright holder.

Disclaimer and Terms of Use: The Author and Publisher has strived to be as accurate and complete as possible in the creation of this book, notwithstanding the fact that he does not warrant or represent at any time that the contents within are accurate due to the rapidly changing nature of the Internet. While all attempts have been made to verify information provided in this publication, the Author and Publisher assumes no responsibility for errors, omissions, or contrary interpretation of the subject matter herein. Any perceived slights of specific persons, peoples, or organizations are unintentional. In practical advice books, like anything else in life, there are no guarantees of income made. This book is not intended for use as a source of legal, business, accounting or financial advice. All readers are advised to seek services of competent professionals in legal, business, accounting, and finance field.

First Printing, 2016

MEDICAL DISCLAIMER

The information in this book is not intended to replace professional medical supervision. The information in this book is highly effective and it will definitely reduce the physical and mental health complaints of nearly every person, who earnestly uses the herbs and techniques outlined within. In some cases a cure may take place; however, there is no guarantee that physical ailments will be completely cured. Prior to reducing or stopping allopathic medications, do consult with a qualified physician.

Free Gifts

Bonus #1 – Grab Free Books!!!!!!!!

As a way of saying thank you for downloading this book I would like to give you two free books, which are available exclusively for my readers. The free book "Juicing for Health – 35 Juicing Recipes for Everyday Health Problems", is packed full of useful healthy juice recipes and Success Hacks - 31 Mind-Set Hacks to Increase Productivity and Career Success, is packed full of helpful mind hacks for developing a more dynamic and enjoyable lifestyle!

Introduction

Do you suffer with gut health problems?
Do you feel bloated after you eat?
Do you find it impossible to lose weight?
Do you suffer with food allergies?
Do you suffer with constipation/diarrhoea?
Do you suffer with acid reflux?
Do you suffer with a dull stomach ache?
Do you suffer with feelings of nausea?

If you regularly suffer from some of these symptoms, then chances are that you have some gut health issues. How many people suffer with one or other form of gut health issues?...Probably the majority of people in one way or another, or at least some of the time, after all who hasn't ate too much Sunday roast or Christmas dinner?

But when these issues become noticeable, on a regular basis and they start to take over your life to the degree that you have to make many special changes in your lifestyle, in order to accommodate them, well that's when things become intolerable. Sadly western medicine isn't a whole lot of help here. Your average GP will recommend an antacid or possibly some enzymes and some general health advice and that's about that, other than that you're on your own!

However, there is light at the end of the tunnel, you don't have to suffer with unruly gut health issues anymore!

In this book we shall take an overview of gut health issues and then provide a wide range of advice regarding foods, supplements and general health advice, in order to get your life back on track. If you follow the advice therein, you will either find a complete resolution to your gut health issues or at the very least, you will at last have a handle on how to deal more effectively with your gut health problems, with a significant reduction in irksome gut health symptoms!

Chapter One – Why is your Gut in Such a Mess!!!

There is a certain amount of genetics involved in gut health issues, but by and large gut health issues come about as a result of lifestyle and diet.

From a genetic point of view celiac disease (whereby the body cannot absorb gluten from grains) has a strong genetic disposition. However, a lot of people who display gluten intolerance symptoms have developed their condition largely as a result of lifestyle and diet imbalances, rather than hereditary conditions. Recent research has labelled a new variation on this theme called **Non Celiac Gluten Sensitivity** (NCGS).[1] The good news about this research is that it indicates a negative reaction to gluten but without the severity of a celiac condition. What this indicates, is that for individuals who have developed NCGS, chances are that they can largely recover from this condition, whereas genuine full-blown Celiac's usually have to live permanently with a strong gluten intolerance.

Looking back at lifestyle and how it creates most gut problems, I think it is fairly easy to realise that our sedentary lifestyle combined with a poor diet, particularly a diet which is high in processed and denatured foods, results in many health imbalances and gut imbalances are amongst the most common health imbalances.

The reason why gut health issues are so prevalent is because the stomach/gut region is central to digestion in our bodies and digestion determines health. For example, back in the early part of the twentieth century an epidemic disease broke out amongst penitentiaries and asylums in the USA which was labelled "Pellagra". Pellagra resulted in serious health problems and sometimes in death and it turned out that it came about as a result of deficient amino acids in the diets of the inmates. While it gave the appearance of a sort of plague, once a healthy diet was implemented all symptoms rapidly disappeared!

So digestion is vital for health and we largely forget this. When we think about digestive health, we tend to think in term of our stomachs as the sole means of digestion and our intestines as been some sort of waste evacuation system. But in reality our stomachs simply predigest our food. On average food which enters the stomach will exit within about 20 minutes. Food has already been pre-digested to a small degree via the enzymes in our saliva. When it goes into the stomach, the hydrochloric acid in our stomachs will then break down this food further so that we now have a soup like semi liquid called "Chyme". Up till now all that has been happening is predigesting, as in chewing with our teeth and melting the food down in our stomachs, does not provide any nutrients but rather it makes the chyme ready to be absorbed in the small intestines.

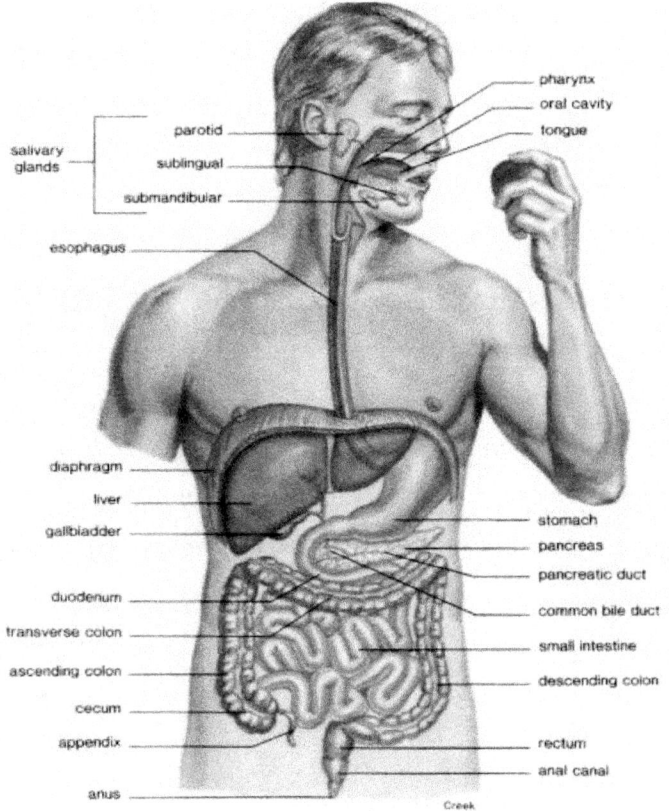

The small intestines are where it's at. In the small intestines, which is misleading as our small intestines are approximately 7 meters or 23 feet in length. It's the intestines which actually absorb the nutrients. Not only are the intestines long but also the intestines containing microvilli, which are small structures which allow for greater absorption of food.

Microvilli – Microscopic structures inside the folds of the small intestines which further enhance the absorbable surface area of the intestines – thus greatly enhancing digestion – many gut imbalances (such as celiac disease for example) impair the microvilli's capacity to absorb nutrients, which in turn results in a wide range of infirmities – remember your only as healthy as your body's ability to absorb nutrients and thus prevent malnutrition from taking place!

So absorbing the nutrients form our food is a complicated and time consuming effort. Some food travels quickly through the intestines, but depending upon genetic makeup and the kinds of food which we are eating, it can take up to several days to fully absorb nutrients from our food.

What is the cause of ill-health in most cases?

Usually the cause of ill-health can be traced back in some way to malnutrition. Now you might be eating enough food, or even more than enough food, but if the food is highly processed and denatured, the net result is malnutrition which can kick of a wide variety of chronic forms of ill health. Once the body struggles to maintain a homeostatic balance, one of the first lines of defence to take a hit is the digestive system, which means either the stomach and/ or the intestines.

One common form of imbalance is food allergies, such as gluten intolerance for example. But also most people have one or more allergic responses to different foods, which are in and of itself an indicator of imbalance. If the stomach is doing its job of predigestion effectively and the small intestines are doing their job of food absorption and elimination of toxins effectively, then most allergic responses will be nullified. Food allergies tend to indicate either a genetic predisposition towards intolerance, to a particular food, or an imbalance in the digestive system.

Some Common Stomach/Gut Health Conditions Causes

There are lots of stomach/gut health conditions which come about as a result of this imbalance.

NCGS (Non Celiac Gluten Sensitivity): As noted earlier many people who have a gluten problem, have developed it as a consequence of a stomach/gut digestive system which is out of balance.

Acid Reflux: Allopathic medicine would have you believe that your acid reflux symptoms have come about as a consequence of irregular acid activity, within the stomach, which results in acid moving from the stomach out into the oesophagus, with painful consequences. The allopathic solution is to give the patient an antacid, which settles the stomach by adding in a base to balance out the acid. However, complementary medicine suggests that acid reflux is created by too little acid in the stomach, which results in an imbalance whereby stomach acid comes about in spits and spurts and some of this makes its way to the oesophagus.

Nausea: Feeling nauseous is very common for pregnant ladies and people who are feel car or sea sick, but some people feel nauseous for no apparent reason, or as a reaction to either smelling or eating certain food. Western medicine has no solution for this other than suggesting an anti-emetic. However from a complementary health perspective, nausea is created by an energetic imbalance in the stomach. In Traditional Chinese Medicine (TCM) there are several energetic meridians in the body, and two of them (the stomach and spleen meridians) directly affect the stomach and can cause nauseous symptoms if unbalanced. Usually the imbalance will come about from poor dietary habits.

Stomach Ache: There are several causes of stomach ache which includes irritable bowel syndrome (IBS), which is again causes by a stomach imbalance; sudden cramping pains (often caused by constipation whereby food does not digest in the intestines and instead it backs up and creates pressure on the stomach), a dull ache caused by an imbalance of healthy bacteria in the gut, which results in discomfort and a vague sense of stomach upset; bacterial infection which can include stomach ulcers (which are also caused by bacterial infection), which usually results from a lack of health bacteria in the gut. If you suddenly suffer from intense stomach ache, check it out with your doctor as there are some serious health conditions which involve stomach pain, but nine times out of ten stomach aches come about as a result of a stomach/gut imbalance.

Constipation/Diarrhoea: Although appearing as the polar opposites constipation (the inability to defecate) and diarrhoea (too much defecation), are often interlinked and it is not uncommon for individuals to flip around from constipation to diarrhoea and back again.

Constipation usually comes about either because of a poor diet, often a low fibre diet, and/or stomach/gut imbalances, whereby the digestive system becomes incapable of effectively digesting the food.

Diarrheal tends to come about as a result of an unbalanced digestive system whereby the body, in an effort to maintain homeostasis, suddenly evacuates waste products from the gut. We can also see how in some cases the body can flip back and forth between constipation and diarrhoea. Now in some cases, in advanced old age the digestive system is wearing down due to age and this can result in this condition, but other than advanced age the body should not be doing this. So in most cases constipation and diarrhoea are a sign of imbalance.

Leaky Gut Syndrome: Leaky Gut Syndrome is the new syndrome on the block! It's easy to label our health by saying I have IBS or I have Leaky gut Syndrome etc., but what we must remember is that allopathic medicine likes to label a bunch of symptoms according to a blanket label. According to allopathic medicine, leaky gut syndrome takes place when toxins which should be effective dealt with in the intestines, end up been released back into the bloodstream with a lot of negative health effects. Now while this situation is genuine, what is the cause?

Leaky gut syndrome is again another sign that there is a serious imbalance in your digestive health. Western medicine likes to label symptoms and then promote pharmaceutical treatments, but really most of these conditions can be reversed by simply getting your stomach and gut to rebalance and go back to working effectively and leaky gut syndrome is one such condition.

So to summarise while genetics plays a part, by and large most stomach and gut problems are as a direct consequence of lifestyle and diet and can be effectively reversed with some changes in these areas or at least the symptoms can be reduced greatly if not completely reversed. In the next two chapters we will cover foods which should be avoided and lifestyle changes which should be made followed by some great supplements, which will greatly help to restore this stomach/gut balance!

Footnotes

1. J Am Cull Nutr. 2014;33(1):39-54. doi: 10.1080/07315724.2014.869996.

Non-celiac gluten sensitivity: literature review.

Mansueto P[1], Seidita A, D'Alcamo A, Carroccio A.

[1]a Internal Medicine, University Hospital of Palermo , Palermo , ITALY.

Chapter Two – Good Habits for Everyone to Follow

In the next chapter we will get into some strategies for dealing with specific stomach/gut imbalances, but prior to doing so let's take a quick look at the basics of healthy stomach/gut maintenance.

Simple Food Advice

Probably the single biggest factor which causes an unbalanced gut is diet. I think we all know about this but it can be difficult to change our diet. However, at least we have to try and be sensible. Just take a trip down to your local supermarket/minimarket and have a look around at most of the foodstuffs present therein. If you try to take an objective look at what you see, rather than simply reacting out of habit, you will notice that around 80% of the food available is either junk (as in biscuits, cakes, ice creams, sodas and so forth), or it might as well be junk as in its highly processed foods. For example most cereals and breads are highly processed as too are dairy products. Fish is usually okish, so long as it's not salmon (as farmed salmon is often high in toxins) or canned fish.

Meat on the other hand is a veritable war zone of injected hormones and chemicals, so most of this is also junk. So what you are left with is the vegetables and fruits, most of which has been over fertilised and often picked and frozen, shipped half way around the world and stored in freezer for an indeterminate period of time! The average apple available in most American super markets, for example, will be up to six months old!

Fresh orange juice is often made from a pulp, which has a whole bunch of additives mixed in there, and it too has usually been in the deep freeze for a mini-ice age!

And just because it tastes good and appears authentic doesn't mean anything. By and large most foods, even the apparently fresh ones have been processed weeks or even months before we have gotten our hands on them. And even good old organic cannot be trusted. Most organic food is not as organic as you might think. Basically unless you bought it direct from the farm, there is no way to know whether it is really fresh (versus deep frozen for a period of time) or that it really is organic!

I'm not saying this to depress you, after all I also buy food from my local supermarket, and unless you live in a region surrounded by organic farmers, where you can buy produce direct from them or you have big cash reserves, whereby you can buy the highest quality food from a top quality health food store, then you just have to get on with eating a bunch of denatured food!

However, while it is virtually impossible these days to have access to the best quality food, at least we can try and steer things into the right direction. For example, if you have a farmers market near you, try and buy fruits and vegetables there. There is a good chance that the food is not organic but there is a good chance that it's actually fairly fresh. Try and buy organic fruit and vegetables from trusted sources, if you can find them. Also wash both fruit and vegetables thoroughly, so as to get some of the chemicals of off them prior to eating them and finally have a look at your eating habits and try to reduce dependence on processed foods where possible.

While it would be ideal to live on an organic farm and eat everything fresh from Mother Nature, this is probably not going to be the reality for most of us.

However, I do believe that even if the food isn't organic and it's probably deep frozen etc., that at least where most of our food intake is home prepared instead of out of a bag or a box, that chances are that it's reasonably healthy. Try where possible to eat as much fruit and vegetables as you can and try to eat raw where possible. As raw food, especially raw vegetables and fruits are high in enzymes (at least some of the time depending upon deep freezing etc.). So at least when we prepare our own food, we are not adding in a bunch of preservatives and additives.

The thing to remember with the modern food industry is that it's all about making money and the way to do this is to make everything appear fresh even if it's not. Think about it this way, if you go into your local store and you buy a fruit or a vegetable that's out of season, then how can it be available unless it has been deep frozen? If you buy a fruit or vegetable, which isn't readily available in your country, then it has been picked from some other country and usually shipped over, in which case it's many weeks or months old!

So one simple way to try and maintain a healthy diet, is to try to eat food according to season, because chances are that if it's in season, then there is a good chance that its actually fresh!

Another thing with the food industry is of course preservatives and additives, so that all those nice tasty foods present in jars, tins, packets and bags are all nice and fresh, many months after they are purchased. So keeping them fresh artificially is good for business, but it's bad for the consumer as we take this crap into our body's, over time toxins build up which make it difficult for our gut to cope with them!

So following on from the old adage that prevention is the best cure, try where possible to eat organic, ideally from the farm and even if this is not possible, try your best to tip the balance over towards eating foods, which are home prepared rather than highly processed, regardless how good they taste.

Finally if we take a look at sources of macronutrients, namely proteins, carbohydrates and fats, we have to take a look at how we are getting these micronutrients. For example in many western countries, huge amounts of bread and dairy products have been the mainstay of diets for centuries. However, most bread today, for example, isn't what it used to be rather it's usually full of cheap starches, even if it appears to be multi-grain, often the multi-grain is more or less a cosmetic after thought. Just make some brown bread at home and compare it to multi-grain, from your local shop, and see how you feel after five or six slices of each and you will notice some discomfort and bloating with the supermarket multi-grain versus homemade. I know that everyone cannot bake their own bread and that supermarket multi-grain, is far better than supermarket white bread, but it's still not great.

Dairy is also questionable, since it's heavily processed versus raw milk and dairy products which have been made on the farm. So I know it can be difficult or even impossible to change these things, but at least we should reduce our dependency upon them. For example, growing up in Ireland, vast quantities of white bread, cheese, processed milk and endless cereals was the name of the game and this is a recipe for gut problems. Because processed bread is starchy, milk and dairy products are full of lactose (unless you are using raw milk which can be hard to get your hands on). So even if you cannot stop taking these foodstuffs, at least reduce your dependency on them.

When I was growing up about 75% of all the food, which I was eating, could be classified under these groups and this sort of highly processed food, combined with a lack of fruit and vegetables in the diet will result in gut problems!

Also in Asian countries rice is very popular which is fine. But rice up to about 60 years ago was heavy organic rice, which was yellow in colour and had a thick outer husk, which is highly nutritious. But modern processed rice has been denatured, in the same way that processed white sugar has been denatured. They have thrown out the outer husk and what you left with as a highly polished, tasty and fairly un-nutritious white grain. It looks pretty but it's not that healthy. So where possible go for organic rice, but most organic rice isn't even really organic. But at least you can reduce your dependency on rice. These days I live in India and a lot of pole in South India eat pounds of rice per day, which is too much. Many of them have distended stomachs, because just like beer drinkers in the west develop stomach distension, so too do many Asian people develop stomach distension.

I'm not suggesting that you give up your favourite foods, but just realise that different cultures have developed a dependence upon certain kinds of food, which has come about historically. But these foods are not the same food which we are using today, so for a start bread, dairy, rice and other cereals where far healthier pre-world war II. Secondly, we tend to eat more foods these days and thirdly we are less active than we sued to be. So because grandpa used to eat a truck load of bread and dairy 60 years ago, when the food was all organic and he worked doing physical labour on the farm for 10 hours a day, whereby his body was like a furnace and burnt off all of the carbohydrates and calories, so of course he was healthy. But now we are eating the same food while leaving a sedentary lifestyle, eating denatured food and lots of it!

Consequently we have to change some of our historical eating patterns, because for a start we don't need such a volume of food. Back in the old days a farmer or manual labourer could easily eat a 1000 grams of carbohydrates a day and burn it off, because they needed 5000 plus calories a day, because of psychical work. If you are a sedentary office worker, then chances are that you will only need somewhere between 2000 to 3000 calories of total food per day, depending upon gender and physical side and general activity levels. So we have to take a look at our food habits and make some changes.

Also because so much of these stable food items are now just junk, probably the easiest way to relieve our digestive systems is to get a little built creative and try to eat a variety of foods, so as to give our gut a chance. If we're eating a pound of bread a day or two pounds of rice a day or a pound of cereals per day or a pound of cheese and other dairy products a day, it's just a bit much for our digestive system to deal with. The simplest way to give your digestive system a break, is to give it a variety of foods, ideally in a balanced way which includes vegetables and fruits. Chances are that when we eat a variety of foods, even if these foods are not organic, that we get a better variety of macro and micronutrients and also it puts less pressure on out guts, as eating vast quantities of the one food, requires a lot of the same sort of enzymes to break it down. So when we eat vast quantities of one kind of food, even if organic, it ends up in a backlog of undigested food in our gut and sometimes even the development of an allergy to that kind of food!

General Good Eating Habits

Before taking a look at supplements for people who are having gut problems, we should first of all remind ourselves to check our eating habits, as it's not just the food you eat but also how you eat which is really important. According to hatha yogis we should chew our food 44 times before swallowing!

I know if we all did this, we would be very slim (because we would not be eating much food) and we would have really big lower faces (thanks to our huge masseter muscles), but on a more practical note, we should at least make a point of chewing our food. I remember when I was young, my brother Tony mastered the art of eating and swallowing a full sized McVities digestive biscuit (it's about 2.5 inches in diameter) in one go and while it was entertaining to watch, this is obviously not a good way to eat our food. Yet most of us do something similar most of the time. In our busy society our tendency is to eat our food in gulp like fashion, as if we haven't seen food for several days and had to satisfy our hanger. Another aspect of modern food eating habits is to sit over our food face down and rat like pigs in a through, we gulp our food down as if are in a race to see who finishes first!

Chew Your Food Thoroughly: Well these are all really bad food eating habits. While it may not be practical or even enjoyable to chew our food for 44 times, we should at least be cognizant that we are eating our food and chew it according to texture. Something like oats or rice pudding can be swallowed, without any really chewing as they are already semi-solid in nature, but foods like meat, fish, bread, biscuits etc., should be chewed and broken down into a semi solid, prior to leaving our mouth. Looking at Mother Nature, this is what our salivary glands are for. The idea is to have the saliva break the food down in our mouth so that it is semi-solid, then the stomach acid makes it more liquid, so it become a soup like substance, called chyme and finally this liquid substance filters through the intestines delivering nutrients as it goes.

So the first step to good gut health is good digestion, and this means chewing our food. Gobbling down great big chunks of red meat, for instance, is really putting stress on our gut. If we take a look at a typical western styled lunch of baguette filled with chicken, for example, when we gulp this down bits of chicken and bread are sitting in our stomachs and since the stomach empties its content within about 20 minutes, the chunks of bread and chicken are still only semi-solid. No wonder the intestine gets back logged and this can be particular severe on foods such as red meat, which are notorious for festering inside the intestines and take at least 24 hours to digest and sometimes more. This is also why it is good to take a variety of meats, over the course of a week, as red meat in particular is difficult to digest. Also some vegetarian foods are famously difficult to digest with noodles been slow to digest, for example.

Anyhow the first step to gut health is to watch your diet and the second is to chew your food, so as to give your gut a chance to properly digest it.

Eating and Activity: Another aspect of eating food is activity. These days I see lots of people eating while walking, for instance, which makes no sense at all as it makes digestion difficult. Another thing is eating while sitting at our desk feeling stressed. For a start we are probably bent over our desk which makes digestion difficult and worrying or stressing, while eating is a real no no!

From a Traditional Chinese medical (TCM) point of view, we should eat in a relaxed and conscious manner, we should be aware that we are eating and enjoy and feel the nurturing effects, as this boosts both yang (active) and ying (nurturing) energy. While this sounds esoteric, it is in fact a very common sense approach to eating, as conscious awareness helps us to relax, which in turn will relax our digestive system; also we will eat more slowly thus allowing our digestive enzymes and stomach acid to do their work and we will feel more contented, which in turn will make us less likely to eat too much. Often times when we rush through our food, we don't even notice that we are eating and end up eating more. Have you ever ate an ice cream or a chocolate bar, only to find out that the last bite was the tastiest and you wish you had more? Chances are you gobbled down the treat so quickly, that you only consciously noticed that you were eating chocolate or ice cream, when you imbibed your last mouth full!

Water Intake At Mealtime: Other good food device is to watch our water intake prior to and post food intake. Our stomach is an acid bath and if we drink water either just before or just after food, we end up diluting the acid, which in turn limits the digestibility of the food. You can of course take milk or other beverages, as they will either be acids or bases, but don't take water with your meal as its ph. neutral so it will put the stomach of!

Another good piece of eating advice is to eat less rather than more. In Japan, for example, the people of the Islands of Okinawa are famous for their longevity. There are several factors, which help them live such a long life, but one of the major factors recognised is that they eat until they are still slightly hungry. The brain takes 15 minutes to catch up with the stomach, so if you stop eating when you are full, about 15 minutes later you will feel really bloated! So there is some real wisdom in the Okinawans approach to eating!

Who hasn't eaten too much food at Christmas, thanksgiving or at a birthday party or in a restaurant while on holidays, but let's be honest is it good for health?

Certainly not, as lying on our bed feeling like a beached whale, for a few hours, is not a pleasant way to spend our afternoon or evening and think about the damage which is been done to our gut. The food is simply backing up and been undigested thus making the entire digestive system run badly. You can do it now and again and get away with it, but if you repeatedly abuse your gut, it will bite back with a variety of gut health issues!

Avoid Spicy Food: Another good piece of advice is to avoid very spicy foods. I know some people love eating spicy food, but spicy food especially if mixed with hard liquor is a recipe for disaster, as it will mess up your stomach! Also another consideration is to balance spicy with non-spicy. In India, for example, spicy food is popular, but so is eating rice mixed with curd (natural yoghurt) at the end of the meal. The thing about natural yoghurt, is that it is a base and it neutralises the acidic effects of spice. So yoghurt or milk are good foods to help wash down a spicy meal, and whatever you do don't drink water when eating spicy food. You Tube is full of entries of people swallowing hot chilli's and then trying to recover by drinking water, well water actually reignites the spice and makes things worse! Next time you eat something too spicy at the restaurant, order a glass or milk or natural yoghurt and forget about the water as it will do more harm than good!

Eat Frequently: Eating frequently is another good protocol. Although most of us like to binge these days, our bodies actually like to eat little but often. Although this can vary from person to person, as some people do better on fewer meals, for the majority of people eating little but often makes the digestive system run well, it helps to maintain metabolic levels and keep nutrients running around the body.

Don't eat late at night. Back in Ireland it's a popular past time for many people go to the pub and drink alcohol, followed by the inevitable take away as beer encourages appetite. But this is a disastrous decision, as one pint of beer contains around 200 calories, so say 4 pints of beer equals 800 calories, all of which are carbohydrates. Then add in another 1500 calories, in the form of a burger, french fries and a bottle of coke and you are now looking at a days' worth of calories followed by sleep!

This is a crazy idea as the liver goes asleep at around 10pm in the evening. Large intakes of calories, just before sleep, will bloat you while you sleep and leave you hungry when you wake up, for the food hasn't been processed. Then when you wake up, you eat more which encourages weight gain and a backlog of food in the intestines!

The same also goes for non-drinkers. Say you work night shift, well don't come home at 5am and eat a big meal and then sleep, rather eat something small and have a really big meal when you wake up, it will work out far better for your body. The human body is designed to process food during daylight hours, so try as best you can to keep most of you're eating between 6am and 6pm where possible, at a push you can still eat till around 9pm at night, but definitely eating later than that is a serious no no for most people's digestive systems!

Hydrate: Finally back to water again, do drink enough water, as in at least 1 litter (2 pints) a day, and this could be as high as 10 litters (20 pints) depending upon climate. While some people suggest that water is not important, actually it is.

Have you ever felt thirsty after a meal? Well the reason why is because digestion uses water, if you want to digest your food you have to drink water. The best policy is to sip water throughout the day. Also carbohydrates suck in water. Every gram of carbohydrates brings along 4 grams of water along with it, so if you are eating a lot, you have to take in a lot of water, otherwise the body will become dehydrated!

Chapter Three – Common Gut Health Problems and How to Treat Them

Ok so say you have some gut health issues and you want to improve things, so what should you do about it?

Well first of all follow the advice listed above. Get your diet in order and do all the right things, like eating little but often, chewing your food, varying your food, eating a healthy diet etc. But this is simply the basics, as without this no other strategy or supplement will help, if you are eating the wrong things at the wrong times.

So what else can you do to boost gut health?

Well you can start by taking in some gut health orientated food, such as the following.

Good for Gut Health

Ginger: Ginger is a popular food supplement, but also it is a wondrous herb which has many great traits one of which is on digestion. In a clinical study on the effectiveness of ginger on speeding up the breakdown of food in the stomach, they took 24 participants and gave them 1.2grams of ginger one hour prior to eating a meal and then observed how long it took for the food to transit from the stomach into the intestines. Normally it will take approximately 20 minutes for the food to transit, however the average figure which came back in this group was a transit time of only 13 minutes. 1 This indicates that the ginger helped the food predigest approximately 50% faster than normal. What this suggests is that ginger will help food to predigest, which will in turn make for better chyme and thus an easier time on the intestines when it comes to absorbing the food.

Furthermore ginger also helps relieve symptoms of nausea. In another clinical trial on 32 pregnant ladies, who were suffering with morning sickness, they were given 1 gram of ginger per day and by the end of the study 28 out of the 32 women noticed a significant reduction in morning sickness symptoms![2]

So ginger not only helps to breakdown the food but also it helps to settle the stomach, in cases of people who are prone to stomach upset!

There are lots of ways to take ginger. After all you can add ginger into your cooking, but one very effective and tasty way to take ginger is as a tea.

Ginger Tea

1. Take 250ml of water (8 ounces) and add in several slices of ginger, taken directly from ginger root. Simply take some ginger root (about 3 grams per cup) and peel of the outer layer of skin from one part of it and then cut of several slices. Take these slices and either crush slightly or blend in a mix for a few seconds before adding into the water. Another approach is to pound them slightly in a pewter, as once the ginger is crushed a little, its helpful compounds will be released.
2. Boil the water and leave to simmer for a good 10 to 15 minutes, in order to get the essence of ginger out. When we think about boiling vegetables versus steaming, steaming is always recommended because boiling takes out the nutrients from the vegetables and puts it into the water, whereas steaming does not do this. However, in this case we want the nutrients within the ginger to come out into the water as we are going to drink it!

3. You will know the tea is ready when a distinct ginger aroma is smelt.
4. Put a tablespoon of honey into a cup
5. Take one small lemon or half a medium sized lemon and squeeze into the same cup
6. Strain the now boiled ginger water into the cup which has honey and lemon present. If you have done a good job, the tea should be strong enough to sting your throat a little but, this means that you really have got the essence of ginger with all of its amazing benefits!
7. Other options include adding in cinnamon and cardamom, which not only add taste but also they add enormous national benefits as well.

For more information on the powerful effects of ginger and other great herbs, check out my book

"Medicinal herbs"

Peppermint: Peppermint has a calming effect on an upset stomach. It relaxes the muscles of the stomach and helps increase the flow of bile. In particular peppermint has a good effect on symptoms of nausea. In a study on the effects of peppermint on post-operative nausea found that peppermint made a significant improvement in nauseas symptoms in patients who took it.3

Furthermore, peppermint helps relieve irritable bowel syndrome (IBS), due to its ability to relax the intestinal walls. Peppermints ability to relax gastrointestinal muscles, means that it is a good way to treat stomach aches, nausea and constipation.

Regarding dosing peppermint is usually taken as a tea and peppermint tea is commonly found in many health food stores and even supermarkets. Of course you can always make your own peppermint tea as follows;

Peppermint Tea

1. Boil water
2. Add in some peppermint leaves
3. Boil for 10 minutes
4. Strain and serve

Wheatgrass: Wheatgrass is awesome yet underrated herb which can really help gut health. Wheatgrass is simply the grass which becomes wheat, being chopped when the grass is only 6 inches in height. Anyway this grass possesses many amazing benefits which include the following benefits:

- Balances the body's Ph. Levels
- Deoxygenates our bodies
- Protects against cancer
- Boosts red blood cell count
- Cleanses the blood
- Liver detoxification
- Improves digestion
- Extremely high in nutrients including vitamins A, B6, C, K and E, manganese, selenium, copper and zinc
- Very high in dietary fibre
- Thyroid stimulation
- Promotes weight loss
- Strengthens bones
- Regulates blood sugar levels
- Improves blood lipid levels
- Increases athletic performance

Wheatgrass is so potent that it's worth taking as a great health booster and everyone should really take it for a couple of reasons. First of all our diet is very acidic these days, as foods such as cereals, milk and dairy products are all acidic.

Most foods which are bases are vegetables, so unless you are eating a truck load of vegetables, your body is probably going to be too acidic. Our bodies are meant to operate slightly into the base range of around 7.35-7.45. The Ph. Scale runs from 0 to 6 which is most acidic to least acidic, with coke and coffee being around 4, on this scale and then we have water which is Ph. Neutral, which is 7 and then we go from 8, which is least base, to 14 which is most base. So our bodies are meant to be slightly base. Our bloodstream has to maintain this narrow range of 7.35 to 7.45, and in order to maintain this level our body will even bleach minerals out of our bones, in an effort to maintain this narrow range in our bloodstream!

Now aside from immanent death, which would happen if our bloodstreams Ph. levels ran outside of this narrow range, even when our body manages to artificially maintain this blood level balance, the body in general is too acidic and in extreme cases this can result in acidosis, where a variety of complaints can arise which includes:

- Fatigue
- Drowsiness
- Shortness of breath
- Headaches
- Confusion
- Tremors

If you have some of these symptoms, then chances are that you either have acidosis or are on the way there. Few people develop full-blown acidosis, but lots of people suffer from borderline acidosis whereby they have aches and pains, feel fatigued and drained and generally their bodies are not working well.

So what has this got to do with gut issues?

Well while gut Ph. level has to be acidic, the body in general should be base, in order to function efficiently. For example, an acidic environment promotes fungal growth, bacterial growth and viral growth, within the body. When we get our Ph. Levels back into the normal range, this bodily environment isn't suitable for funguses, bacteria or viruses. So getting rid of these pathogenic invaders helps amongst other things a healthy gut. The great thing with wheatgrass is that it helps to get the Ph.levels back inline without resorting to eating large quantities of vegetables each day..

Also wheatgrass is high in fructans which promote lactobacilli (healthy gut bacteria – which aid digestion and help to kill of nasty funguses such as Candida, for example) and they also help promote reabsorption of calcium, which promotes bones health, lowers triglyceride levels, which aids heart health and helps to reduce blood glucose levels.

Another great benefit of wheatgrass is its high micronutrient level, which promotes once again digestive health and finally wheatgrass is very high in soluble fibre, to the degree that ingesting wheatgrass can promote bowel movements, especially in people who are having gut health issues.

Wheatgrass is a great herb and will boost your health in general, but certainly it has a great benefit on gut health. Importantly when you initially take wheatgrass, usually it will have as strong effect on bowel movements. So when you start taking wheatgrass at first, don't be surprised if you end up suddenly having to go to the toilet. Fortunately this will right itself within a few days or weeks. The good news however, is that its' your gut righting itself and the reason why there are so many bowel movements is because the wheatgrass is moving stubborn blockages within the intestines. So getting as this 'crap' (literarily) gets thrown out of our bodies, which is really good for health and most people, who have gut health issues, nearly always there will be a backlog, so moving this backlog is the first step towards good gut health. Also for people who are suffering with diarrhoea, wheatgrass will help to balance the healthy gut bacteria which will have the reverse effect of normalising bowel movements!

Regarding how to take wheatgrass, ideally you should grow your own, but this tends to be a big hassle, so while the organic, made at home in your garden wheatgrass is the best, even still the powder form which you get in your local health store, is still pretty good and well worth your while to take it.

To take wheatgrass in powder form, just take two tablespoons (30 grams) of it and add in around 250 ml (8 ounces) of water, stir with a spoon and drink. If you have been having lots of stomach health issues, then take this 3 times a day initially, but when things settle down, take just once a day, as this is enough to greatly promote gut health and health in general!

Apple Cider Vinegar:

Apple Cider Vinegar (ACV) goes hand in hand with wheatgrass in that it is a powerful general health elixir and also it is very good for gut health. The benefits of ACV includes the following:

- Balances the bodies Ph. Levels
- Promotes digestion and stomach health
- Aids blood circulation
- Aids weight loss
- Good for heart health
- Relieves joint pain
- Anti-cancerous

Now out of all these great effects, form the point of view of gut health we are interested in ACV because of its Ph. balancing effects and also because of its effects on balancing stomach health.

There are two factors worth considering here. Firstly, ACV helps to balance the acidic levels within the stomach. Acid reflux is seen as an imbalance in the stomach, whereby acid spurts up from the stomach into the oesophagus thus creating heart burn. However, from a holistic point of view, acid reflux is not caused by erratic acid activity, but rather it is caused by insufficient stomach acid levels. Where ACV helps is that it balances the Ph. environment in the stomach, thus helping to normalise stomach acidic activity. So even though ACV, like wheatgrass acts as a base on the body, however ACV is actually an acid, so while it converts into a base after digestion, prior to digestion it is acidic and it helps the stomach balance its acid levels!

The second advantage is that it works while promoting an acidic environment in the stomach which encourages lactobacilli, which are helpful bacteria which thrive in an acidic environment and help to maintain a healthy gut and help to kill off gut fungi such as Candida!

ACV is very easy to take, simply take one tablespoon of ACV in a glass and add in 250ml (8ounces) of water, stir with a spoon and drink. The only thing to watch out for with ACV is that it is acidic, so make sure you wash your teeth by rinsing your mouth out with some water or another beverage afterwards, so as to wash away the acidic deposits from the teeth. Other than that ACV is easy to take although it is bitter in taste. Also the ideal ACV is slightly smoky in colour because it possesses a string of material known as 'the mother' which is very potent. So when buying ACV try and get the version of ACV which is a little bit misty in colour.

ACV will have a general balancing effect on gut health and is really helpful for people who suffer with acid reflux problems. However, it's not the sort of supplement which you take when you have acute acid reflux symptoms. When you are suffering from acid reflux and you want to treat the symptom take an antacid, natural yoghurt or milk. But get into the habit of taking at least one glass a day of ACV and over a period of a few weeks it will have an impact on stomach acid and gut health in general.

Also ACV goes really well with wheatgrass. I find that washing down a glass of ACV with a glass of wheatgrass is a good way to get my daily quota of both and of course the wheatgrass washes of the acidic ACV deposits form my teeth as wheatgrass is a base.

Take a look at a video here where we show you how to prepare ACV and wheatgrass for health

How to take wheatgrass and (ACV)

Kombucha: Kombucha is a popular health drink, which is basically a sugary black tea, which after fermentation it becomes laden with healthy bacteria, vinegar, b vitamins, probiotics, enzymes and healthy acids (acetic, lactic and gluconic).

Benefits of kombucha includes:

- Gut health
- Weight loss
- Detoxification

- Improved immune system
- Reduced joint pain
- Anti-cancerous

In particular, from the point of view of gut health the really great thing about kombucha is its amazing variety of probiotics which help to keep the digestive process working properly.

Kombucha is high in Acetobacter , Gluconacetobacte, Lactobacillus and Zygosaccharomyces probiotics. So kombucha will go along way towards getting your gut to work well. With so many probiotics these will flush out funguses (such as Candida) and aid in digestion.

Also kombucha is high in free antioxidants, which helps to counteract free radicals in the gut, which also aids digestive health. Kombucha has also been known to treat stomach ulcers and helps both to prevent and treat leaky gut syndrome.

Kombucha is a very powerful gut health tonic and one or two glasses a day, will go along way towards improving stomach and gut health. But do note that there are so many probiotics in kombucha that if your gut is out of balance, that initially kombucha might result in symptoms such as bloatedness, gas, mild stomach ache and diarrhoea. Don't' worry about this, as it is the guts way of normalising under the powerful and potent impact of kombucha. So when you start taking kombuhca, ease into it by taking one glass a day for a few days and then build up to two or three glasses a day, then after a few weeks when you feel things settle down, then reduce back to a maintenance level, of one glass a day.

Kefir: Kefir is a Turkish cultured dairy product, which is very high in probiotics. Kefir has been used as a health food for centuries and amongst its many benefits are:

- Improves immunity levels
- Heals gut problems
- Helps digest lactose
- Kills of Candida fungus
- Treats allergies
- Strengthens bones
- Detoxicant

Kefir's many benefits come from its nutrient rich make-up. Kefir is high in vitamin B12, vitamin K2, calcium, biotin, folate, probiotics and enzymes. In particular enzymes and probiotics make kefir a very potent gut health food.

Enzymes reduce once one reaches 30 years of age, which in turn makes it more difficult to digest food, so eating a supplement which is high in digestive enzymes is a great way of improving digestion. Secondly probiotics are healthy bacteria and healthy bacteria fight of nasty digestive fungus's such as Candida, for example.

Kefir is jam packed with probiotics which includes Bifidobacteria, Acetobacter, Lactobacillus Acidophilus, Lactobacillus Bulgaricus, Lactobacillus Caucasus, Lactobacillus Rhamnosus, Lactobacillus and Leuconostoc.

The result of this is that kefir can heal many gut issues include Leaky Gut Syndrome. Also, interestingly it helps people who suffer from lactose intolerance to actually start absorbing lactose!

For anyone who is suffering from gut health issues kefir is worth trying out. However, kefir being a dairy product, it might be difficult to take for anyone who is lactose intolerant. People who suffer with Candida, for example, are lactose intolerant, so they won't initially be able to absorb kefir. In this case it makes more sense to make an effort to detoxify and clean up the digestive system in the first place. So take other supplements such as wheatgrass, ACV and ginger for a while and then slowly add in the kefir.

Moringa: Moringa is a tree which grows well in Southeast Asia, and is often referred to as the "miracle tree" because it is very high in nutrients which includes beta carotene, Vitamin C, carotene and protein. Moringa is so high in nutrients that it has 12 times more vitamin C than an oranges, it has 10 times more vitamin A than carrots and 17 times more calcium than milk, for example!

From the point of view of gut health moringa can help in several ways. For a start moringa is high in antioxidants, which helps to detox the intestines. Secondly, moringa helps to reduce inflammation in the body. Inflammation is the body's way of coping with imbalances in the body; it's a sort of cordon whereby the body cordons off infected areas. For a short time it works well, but after a while chronic health develops. Inflammation in the gut is a real bad thing, as it makes food nutrients absorption difficult and also excretion of wastes difficult. So moringa can help to reduce inflammation through the body, which includes the gut. Also moringa boosts liver functioning, which helps to detoxify the system, which is good as where there is a dysfunctional gut, there will be a buildup of toxins in the body.

Moringa leafs can be used with your meals as in a salad or in a juice, for example. If you cannot get your hands on raw moringa, you can probable get a hold of organic cold – pressed moringa oil. Moringa oil is expensive, but it's potent with about a tablespoonful a day being a really good overall health tonic and of course a gut treatment for gut health problems.

Supplements for Gut Health

So far we have looked at foods which help to cure gut health problems, but there are also some supplements which can help, so let's take a look.

Deglycyrrhizinated licorice (DGL):

Licorice is very good for health and helps cure or improve a wide range of health conditions. However, long-term usage can have a negative impact upon blood pressure levels, oedema and oestrogen levels, thanks to the presence of glycyrrhizin. Whereas deglycyrrhizinated licorice, has all the benefits of licorice but without the potential downsides of glycyrrhizin.

From the point of view of gut health, DGL provides great relief for heartburn, peptic ulcers and gastritis, which relates back to its anti-inflammatory properties and its gut bacteria balancing properties. In a study of 82 patients who took DGL, versus an over the counter peptic ulcer medication, the patients who were given 2 DGL tablets daily, over a period of two years, demonstrated the same level of reoccurrence of peptic ulcers, as the patients who took the peptic ulcer medicine, which suggests that DGL is just as strong as the allopathic medication! [4]

They also note noted in this study that the DGL group, just like the pharmaceutical group, suffered from a big increase in the onset of peptic ulcers after they stopped taking DGL. This suggests that while DGL is as effective as pharmaceutical medications at treating peptic ulcers, it only keeps peptic ulcers at bay, as long as it was taken. So for some people who suffer extreme stomach issues, such as peptic ulcers, DGL will probably end up becoming part of a lifelong treatment plan!

Regarding dosage, usually DGL is taken anywhere from 1 to 3 tablets, at a dosage of 380 to 400mg per tablet. Take the DGL tablet about 30 minutes prior to each meal will help relieve your stomach.

With that in mind, it's important to remember that long-term herbal supplement use can have toxic side effects, just like long-term medications can. With DGL, the majority of the glycyrrhizin has been removed, however, a little still remains, so if you decide to use DGL, over a long period of time, do check your blood pressure, from time to time, and watch out for oedema. Also in some cases liver toxicity can occur. Dglycyrrhizinated licorice, is a great supplement and chances are that there will be no side effects, but this is something to bear in mind for anyone who is on long term medication, and DGL been just as effective as a pharmaceutical drug should be respected as potentially damaging to health, in some cases.

As to why you should use DGL rather than using pharmaceutical drugs, DGL being a natural product will have less side effects, but like any powerful herb, some toxic side effects shall still remain present.

And this is something to remember with the various foods, supplements and health tips mentioned in this book. In an ideal world every health condition would be curable, but in reality gut health can vary from individual to individual. For some people, they will get great relief from their symptoms with a few small changes. Anyone who suffers from a strong food allergy can testify to this! However, for some people no matter how many strategies they try, or foods they take, their gut health issues linger on. For people in this group, the thing to remember is that gut health is a complex topic and although a full-blown cure may not come, certainly with patience and application of good healing strategies, foods and supplements, much relief can be achieved.

So if you have tried everything under the sun and yet still suffer with gut health issues don't despair. Things will get better, but some trial and error may be required, and even if a full recovery does not come, certainly a good improvement can be made. The reason for writing this book is to share some resources with you, which you might not have already considered. While modern health care can help in many ways, there is a tendency to treat patients symptomatically by providing different drugs to treat various symptoms. I'm not saying that complementary health care is better, but what I am saying is that it provides us with some more resources and other options and also that it focuses upon balance, where a rebalance can take place often symptoms will take care of themselves!

Betaine Hydrochloric Acid:

Betaine Hydrochoric Acid is an ideal supplement for people who are suffering from insufficient stomach acid levels. As noted earlier from a complementary point of view, acid reflux is as a direct consequence of deficient stomach acid levels, which result in sporadic production of hydrochloric acid in the stomach, some of which ends up in the oesophagus which results in acid reflux symptoms. Apple Cider Vinegar can help to restore this balance as ACV is an acid, but for more severe cases if ACV doesn't appear to help, it's worth trying out Betaine Hydrochloric Acid.

Betaine HCL will help to rebalance the acid levels in the stomach, which will not only cures acid reflux, but also it help to improve the overall health and vitality of the stomach and gut and finally sufficient levels of HCL are required to effectively breakdown and digest vitamin B12, amino acids and proteins!

Regarding dosage a little bit of trial and error is required. Start by taking a meal which contains at least 20 grams of protein (HCL is required to breakdown the protein). Take 1 Betaine HCL pills (around 650mg) and check in with your stomach, after eating, to see if it has made any difference to digestion. You should feel better, but if you feel a burning sensation chances are that too much acid is been taking. If you feel a burning distension feeling, then reduce down to half a pill. If you feel an improvement or don't feel any improvement, just maintain this one pill per meal and after a couple of days try out 2 pills and see how you feel. Keep experimenting with dosage until you feel an improvement in digestion, but don't feel any discomfort. Once you feel discomfort stop and even reduce dosage a little bit, if need be.

So experiment a little bit, until you are taking enough Betaine HCL, to make a good improvement to digestion, without overdoing it as too much HCL will make you feel ill. For most people the dosing of Betaine HCL shall be somewhere between 3000mg to 5500mg per meal. Taking too little won't do anything to help digestion and taking too much will make for an over acidic gut environment.

Contraindications

One thing which you have to be careful about, when using Betaine HCL, and that is when Betaine HCL is mixed with anti-inflammatory drugs such as aspirin, corticosteroids, Indocin, ibuprofen and NSAIDs (non-steroidal anti-inflammatory drug) in general. The reason is that HCL pills, when mixed into a stomach, which is already containing these drugs can aggravate the stomach lining and even result in bleeding of the stomach lining, or even the development of an ulcer!

So while Betaine HCL is a great way to improve acid reflux and indigestion, you have to be careful otherwise you can make things worse!

Also, anti-inflammatory drugs are very popular, ibuprofen for example (Motrin, Advil, Brofen) is a very popular headache pill, and of course aspirin is very popular, so just check out your medications and don't mix these medications with HCL!

L-glutamine: L-Glutamine is a very useful supplement. L-Glutamine is an amino acid, being the most common amino acid used by the human body (around 30 present of all amino acid nitrogen in the blood is L-Glutamine). Being an amino acid, L-Glutamine will obviously be a big help at building muscle and maintaining lean muscle when dieting, but it also comes with many other benefits which includes:

- L-Glutamine is great for intestinal health, as it helps to rebuild and repair damage to the gut
- It helps to heal ulcers, cure leaky gut syndrome and prevents further damage to the stomach and intestines
- It improves symptoms of Irritable Bowel Syndrome (IBS) and diarrhoea by balancing mucus levels in the stomach lining.5
- Reduces cravings for sweets and alcohol
- Improves the metabolism
- Detoxifies the body (including the intestines)
- Improves blood sugar control
- Anti-cancer agent
- Promotes muscle growth and prevents muscle wasting
- Improves athletic performance and recovery from exercise

So in essence L-Glutamine is a body builder, which in the case of gut issues, it is a body rebuilder, helping to repair gut health issues.

In a study of 20 patients who were fed intravenously for two weeks, they noted that the group, who received L-Glutamine, along with the intravenous food, suffered less gastrointestinal degeneration and demonstrated better permeability than those who didn't. Intravenous feeding has a negative impact upon digestive health, so this study demonstrates the potency of L-Glutamine.6

In another study they noted the healing mechanism of L-Glutamine, whereby it regulates the IgA immune response. IgA is an antibody which fights against bad bacteria and viruses. It also relates to food sensitivities and allergies. So take L-Glutamine will help with food intolerances.7

In yet another study in the Journal of Clinical Immunology they discovered that L-Glutamine regulates the TH2 immune response, which in turn regulates inflammatory cytokines.8 so what this means is that L-Glutamine reduces inflammatory responses, which in turn helps to reduce many gut imbalances.

In summary L-Glutamine can repair damage, reduce food sensitivity and allergic responses and also reduce or even eliminate the inflammatory effect.

L-Glutamine is a must have supplement, for anyone who is facing gut repair issues. Leaky Gut syndrome, for example, isn't just uncomfortable but rather it promotes other degenerative health conditions, such as autoimmune conditions, psoriasis, arthritis and even Hashimotos' disease (a slow thyroid).

When we think about healing gut issues, we have to think in terms of getting rid of toxins, righting imbalances and also repairing organic damage and this is where L-Glutamine comes in handy.

L-Glutamine helps with repairing damage caused by a wide variety of gut health issues including Chrohn's disease, Irritable Bowel Syndrome (IBS), Ulcerative colitis, Diverticulosis and Diverticulitis, for example.

How to Take L-Glutamine

L-Glutamine comes in two forms, which are free form, which has to be taken with food for proper absorption. The other type is known as Trans-Alanyl Glutamine or Alanyl –L - Glutamine. This latter time is more absorbable that free form L-GLutmine, so you can take it on an empty stomach, if you want to. You can take it after your meals and in particular it is helpful either before or after workouts in the gym, as it supports both athletic performance and repair of muscle damage.

Regarding dosage, dosage is usually 2 to 5 grams a day, but up to 10 grams a day can be taken. For people with gut health, it makes most sense to take it three times a day, during mealtime either just before or just after food, so as to help with the digestive process. Also for long-term use it is a good idea to supplement some vitamin B12 every day, which helps to regulate L-Glutamine levels in the body, a sot much L-0Glutamine can result in some toxicity, if too much builds up in the body.

Side effects of too much L-Glutamine includes increased sweating in feet and hands, back pain, joint pain, muscle pain, dizziness, fatigue, headache, runny nose, dry mouth, gas, vomiting and stomach pain. These are unlikely to happen but it's good to know. The vitamin B12 should minimize the tendency of side effects, but if some of these symptoms arise, then reduces dosage accordingly.

Contraindications: L-Glutamine should be avoided for people who are suffering with liver or kidney dysfunction.

Aloe Vera: Aloe Vera is a super plant which has many great benefits which includes:

- High in anti-inflammatory properties

- Helps relieve constipation

- Promotes regular bowel movements

- Detoxification

- Encourages good gut bacteria

- Helps treat leaky gut syndrome

- Helps relieve heartburn/acid reflux

- High in antioxidant and antibacterial properties

- Fights off candida fungus

- Fights off parasitic infections

- Treats mouth ulcers

- Reduces dental plaque

- Improves skin quality

- Prevents wrinkles

So in summary aloe Vera is an amazing plant which demonstrates a wide range of effects. In particular it works wonderfully well on gut health.

Aloe Vera is high in nutrients including calcium, copper, chromium, magnesium, manganese, potassium, sodium, selenium and zinc; It is high in the antioxidant vitamins A, C and E; it is also a great source of vitamin B12, choline and folic acid. Furthermore, aloe Vera contains 8 digestive enzymes (alianase, amylase, alkaline phosphatase, catalase, carboxypeptidase, cellulose, lipase and peroxidase) which help to break down foods. Also, Aloe Vera is high in probiotics (healthy gut bacteria), which help to restore the balance of gut health. In a study on the effect of Aloe Vera on lactobacilli probiotics, they noted a significant increase in levels of L. acidophilus, L. plantarum and L. casei, via aloe vera supplementation.8 Finally Aloe Vera promotes regulation of Ph. Levels throughout the body, which in turn aids gut health.

How to Take Aloe Vera

There is a variety of ways in which you can take aloe Vera. You can take it as a juice or as a capsule. Regarding dosage you can start on a small amount, say 1tsp twice a day taken before meals. Then slowly increase the amount taken up to a maximum of 4 tbsp. twice a day. How much you will take, will vary according to your gut health issues and your reaction to aloe Vera juice or capsules. Aloe Vera promotes bowel movements, so it is a good idea to start of, taken a small amount particularly at first, since it will help to clear any backlog within the intestines, hence too much too soon might result in diarrhoea like symptoms!

Also on the other hand many people avoid aloe Vera, believing it to be a laxative, but actually it is quite safe to take and even kids can take it, but they should take a very small l amount like a tsp. or two per day. Rather aloe Vera is safe but it does rebalance bowel movements and can result in a laxative like effect, if you take too much too soon!

Footnotes

1. Ginger for Nausea and Vomiting in Pregnancy: Randomized, Double-Masked, Placebo-Controlled Trial

VUTYAVANICH, TERAPORN MD, MSC;
KRAISARIN, THEERAJANA MD;
RUANGSRI, RUNG-AROON BSC.

2. Eur J Gastroenterol Hepatol. 2008 May;20(5):436-40. doi: 10.1097/MEG.0b013e3282f4b224.

   Effects of ginger on gastric emptying and motility in healthy humans.

   Wu KL[1], Rayner CK, Chuah SK, Changchien CS, Lu SN, Chiu YC, Chiu KW, Lee CM.

   [1]Division of Hepatogastroenterology, Department of Internal Medicine, College of Medicine, Chang Gung Memorial Hospital, Kaohsiung Medical Center, Chang Gung University, Kaohsiung, Taiwan. kengliang_wu@yahoo.com.tw

3. Peppermint oil: a treatment for postoperative nausea
   Sylvina Tate MSc BSc (Hons) RGN DipN PGDE RNT*
   Article first published online: 28 JUN 2008
   DOI: 10.1046/j.1365-2648.1997.t01-15-00999.x

4. Morgan AG, Pacsoo C, McAdam WA (June 1985). "Maintenance therapy: a two year comparison between Caved-S and cimetidine treatment in the prevention of symptomatic gastric ulcer recurrence." Gut 26 (6): 599-602.

5. HIV Clin Trials. 2003 Sep-Oct;4(5):324-9.

L-glutamine supplementation improves nelfinavir-associated diarrhea in HIV-infected individuals.

Huffman FG[1], Walgren ME.

[1]Department of Dietetics and Nutrition, College of Health and Urban Affairs, Florida International University, Miami, Florida 33172, USA. huffmanf@fiu.edu

6. **Glutamine and the preservation of gut integrity**

R.R.W.J. van der Hulst MD, M.F. von Meyenfeldt MD, N.E.P. Deutz MD, P.B. Soeters MD (Prof), R.J.M. Brummer MD, B.K. von Kreel PhD, J.W. Arends MD (Prof)

Published: 29 May 1993

7. Clin Immunol. 1999 Dec;93(3):294-301.

Effect of glutamine on Th1 and Th2 cytokine responses of human peripheral blood mononuclear cells.

Chang WK[1], Yang KD, Shaio MF.

8. Gut Microbes. 2012 Jan 1; 3(1): 4–14.
   doi: 10.4161/gmic.19320
   PMCID: PMC3337124

   The role of gut microbiota in immune homeostasis and autoimmunity

   Hsin-Jung Wu[1,2,*] and Eric Wu

9. Acta Biomed. 2012 Dec;83(3):183-8.

Effect of Aloe vera juice on growth and activities of Lactobacilli in-vitro.

Nagpal R[1], Kaur V, Kumar M, Marotta F.

Chapter Four - Gut Healing Program

Ok so we have covered a lot of ground here in the previous three chapters. We have learnt about good eating habits, which act as a foundation for good gut health; we have learnt about everyday foods with can help to restore gut health balance and we have also found out about some great supplements to treat specific gut health problems. So how best can we use this information?

First of all take a look at chart one and two, as these two charts spell out for you the areas in which each foodstuff or supplement come into play. Just take a look:

Chart One

Health Foods and their Uses for Treating Gut Health Problems

Gut Health Basics

- Chew Your Food Thoroughly
- Eating and Activity
- Water Intake At Mealtime
- Avoid Spicy Food
- Eat Frequently
- Hydrate

	Ginger	Peppermint	Wheatgrass	ACV	Kombucha	Kefir	Moringa
Detox			x				x
Rebuild							x
Rebalance	x	x	x		x	x	x
Digestion	x	x		x	x	x	x
Acid Reflux				x			
Nausea	x	x					
Stomach Ache		x					
Diarrhoea							
Constipation		x	x				
Anti-Fungal			x		x	x	
Anti-mcirobial			x				
Anti-Parasitic			x				

Chart Two				
Health Supplements and their Uses for Treating Gut Health Problems				
	Deglycyrrhizinated licorice	**Betaine Hydrochloric Acid**	**L-glutamine**	**Aloe Vera**
Detox			x	x
Rebuild	x		x	x
Rebalance	x	x	x	x
Digestion	x	x	x	
Acid Reflux	x	x	x	
Nausea				x
Diarhea			x	x
Constipation			x	x
Anti - Fungal				x
Anti-mcirobial				x
Anti-Parasitic				x

First of all we can see that for any hope of improving our gut health, we must carry out some basics, which are chewing food thoroughly; concentrating while you eat on your eating; avoiding water just before, during and just after eating; avoid spicy food and if you eat spicy food then balance it with a base such as milk or natural yoghurt; eat fairly frequently or at least regularly and stay hydrated. These are the absolute basics. If you think you can take a few herbs and supplements, but abuse your gut by either overeating, underrating, eating the wrong types of foods, or eating erratically at all times of the day and night, then forget about it. Our bodies love regularity, get regular with your eating and eat a balanced diet, is the first step in rebalancing our gut health!

Secondly if we look at chart one, at the various foods which help gut health we can see that these foods (Ginger, Peppermint, Apple Cider Vinegar, Kombucha, Kediri and Moringa) tend to be tonic like in nature. While each one has a slightly different effect, overall the tendency is towards aiding digestion and balancing gut health. Whereas while there are a lot of similarities with the supplements mentioned in chart two (Deglycyrrhizinated licorice, Betaine Hydrochloric Acid, L-glutamine and Aloe Vera) we see that they are more specific in action. Apart from Aloe vera, which is a general tonic, the other supplements are more specific in nature, as in Deglycyrrhizinated licorice, for instance helps stomach acidity, acid reflux and peptic ulcers; Betaine Hydrochoric Acid is great for stomach acidity problems; L-Glutamine is a rebuilder for gut damage.

So putting this altogether we can see that the foods mentioned in chart one should be used as a general tonic, whilst the supplements should be added in to treat more specific problems. For example a person who suffers a lot with acid reflux may take a variety of the helpful foods for stomach problems, but then make a specific point of taking Beltaine Hydrochoric Acid, for low stomach acid levels, deglycyrrhizinated licorice also for balancing stomach acids and L-Glutamine for rebuilding the damaged stomach wall.

The thing is that there is no hard and fast rule as how to take these herbs and supplements. The thing is to try and get a feel for your gut health problem and take herbs and supplements which help with that condition. For example, most people will need to detox there gut, in which case wheatgrass and aloe Vera will be very important. For a person who has stomach acidity problems, for example, they might tend towards taking ginger and peppermint tea and aloe Vera, for example.

So take a look at the herbs and supplements mentioned in this book and use them according to your needs.

The thing to remember with gut health issues is that as noted there are a wide range of possible issues as noted in chapter two. So to rebalance our gut health, we first of all have to make an effort to balance things out and then we have to approach certain symptoms specifically.

Most people will have stomach health issues because they are eating the wrong foods, been physically inactive and also much stressed out. Over time the gut becomes imbalanced. Part of this imbalance is as a consequence of lifestyle and diet and can be readily reversed with lifestyle and diet changes. But more often than not toxins have built up and need to be detoxified. So for most people, the stages of gut rebalancing which have to take place are as follows:

1. Detox
2. Rebalance
3. Rebuild

Detox

For most of us when we develop gut health issues we gather up toxins because the purpose of our gut is to take in food, absorb the nutrients and expel the waste products. When our gut starts going out of balance, we stop absorbing nutrients properly and they also stop excreting properly. On top of this, because much food does not absorb properly, even more toxins build up along the gastrointestinal tract. This increase in toxins can eventually find its way into the bloodstream (Leaky Gut Syndrome) and this can result in the development of chronic ill health. Other things which can take place are over sensitivity to certain food groups and an inability to absorb these particular foods.

In a very healthy gut nearly anything can be eaten, whereas in an unhealthy gut most foods can cause some sensitivity issues. Also once toxins buildup, it becomes a breathing ground for fungus's (such as Candida doe example), viruses and bacterial infections, all of which make things go even further out of balance.

Depending upon the individual, this might result in one person having nauseous symptoms and in another person having diarrhea and in a third person having perhaps gluten sensitivity, for example. Often the outward symptom is a consequence of one's genetic predisposition, so the first step for most people is detox, in order to begin the rebalancing process.

Green Tea: There are various ways to carry out a detox. On one level wheatgrass and Aloe Vera are a really good way to encourage detoxification. Another helpful detox herb is green tea. Green tea is very popular as a healthy tea, but what few people realize is that large quantities of green tea, as in 3 to 5 cups a day, can often greatly help detoxification!

Enema: Enemas are another process encouraged as a way to detox. In the case of an enema, we place a tube inside the anus and pour in saline solution and then go to the toilet. However, while some people love enemas, from my experience enema's only clean out the lower intestine, because at home using an enema bag it's not possible to get the solution up into the small intestines and it's the small intestines which we have to clean. If we use a large quantity of saline water, the net result is an intolerable buildup of pressure, resulting in a sudden evacuation of the bowels. Although the bowel movement might be big, the result is only a cleansing of the lower bowels.

Another approach is to use a laxative. Epsom salts, for example, have a profound effect on clearing out the bowels; all you have to do is to add in one tablespoon into a glass of water and drink it. But Epsom salts works by filling the intestines with a salt which it cannot deal with and so the body draws a huge amount of water into the intestines in order to clear out the salt. Yes it does produce a big result, but then again it dehydrates the body and Epson desalts should not be taken without drinking a lot of water to assist the evacuation process. Also Epson salts can be really aggressive as can other natural laxatives.

Yet another approach is to use colonic irrigation. With colonic irrigation a machine is used to pump a large amount of saline solution through the bowels with the result of a huge evacuation of waste products or the gastrointestinal tract. However, while colonic irrigation is effective it is costly, embarrassing and useless unless you can do with every other week, because the waste products are only sucked out then they refill within a few days. Colonic irrigation can be used in extreme cases of intestinal blockage, which might be required for some people who are suffering from severe constipation, because they are so blocked up that extreme measure sums tube taken. But this in itself is neither a long-term solution nor should it be used habitually. What we have to do is to cleanse the gastrointestinal tract and then once a deep cleanse has ten place we should maintain its balance naturally without the help of enemas, laxatives and colonic irrigation.

In some case blockages are so serious that laxatives are required, but I personally believe in using natural methods, which are more pleasant and more effective. Wheatgrass, for example, if taken several times a day will often promote defecation, especially in someone who suffers with an unbalanced gut. Aloe Vera is also helpful at getting bowel movements going. One of the most effective ways of cleansing the gut is via water therapy.

Water Therapy: Water therapy is very simple, all you have to do is take a large quantity of water within a short period of time and it will flush out the intestines. The traditional approach is to take around 3 liters (5 pints) of water within a period of 30 minutes. However, after trying this method out myself, I can say that it is time consuming and uncomfortable as after the first couple of liters or so, water starts backing up from the stomach into the esophagus and one can even feel a little bit noises. Also, drinking huge quantities of water can in some cases end up diluting the blood, which is very dangerous for health!

Anyway, after trying out this method for a week and feeling all of the above I decided to experiment a little and instead of dinking 3 liters over 30 mints I attempted to drink just 1 liter (1.5 pints) in less than a minute, by taking several big gulps of water. To my surprise and delight I discovered that drinking 1 liter of water, within a minute or so, produced the exact same effect as drinking 3 liters of water over half an hour, and without the nausea and discomfort!

By drinking a smaller quantity of water very quickly I managed to flush out my intestines, as if I had taken a lot more water over a longer period of time. Which leads onto the explanation as to why this methodology is so effective? It works by flushing out ingrained and compacted fecal matter from with the intestinal wall. Remember earlier in chapter 1 there are two diagrams which describe the gastrointestinal system. The second of these two pictures depicts the microvilli. The microvilli are tony convoluted structures found within the wall of the intestines. The small intestines are long (around 20 feet) compared with only 5 feet for the large intestine. The reason being that the greater the surface area of the small intestines, the greater the amount of food absorption which will take place. So on top of being 20 feet long the intestines have an even greater surface area thanks to these microvilli. But on the other hand when gut health becomes compromised, the intestines get blocked and even enemas and laxatives can have difficulty in cleaning out the dirt which is trapped in the microvilli.

This is where water is great. If you ask any geologist he will happily explain how powerful water is at shaping the landscape. Water, the softest of physical objects, over time can clear out the most intransient obstacles!

What I like about water therapy is that it's something which you can do several times a week, every day or even a couple of times a day, if needs be. This means that even the most remote parts of the intestines will get cleared out, over time, and furthermore unlike even efficient methods like colonic irrigation, water therapy can be used frequently, without having to embarrass yourself or spend a lot of money. With water you simply drink a liter of water, in a minute or so, and then when the urge comes to o to the toilet.

Atypically several bladder movements will follow, within the next hour and half and a bowel movement will usually come too. If a bowel movement doesn't come, don't worry about it; it will come in its own time. Keep taking the water therapy, do it twice a day, if you need to, and slowly the blockage will become unblocked.

Also on the other side of the coin, if you try out water therapy and find yourself sitting on the toilet for half of the day, then reduce the volume of water accordingly!

Water therapy is a very natural and non-forceful way of clearing out the intestines and maintaining intestinal health. Also as a final note remember not to take water therapy, if you have to out somewhere within the next hour or so, as the nature of water therapy is that it fills the bladder and intestines with water, and bladder and bowel movements can come along at any time, within that hour and a half period or so.

For a more detailed outline of water therapy and a video on it check out the link below to my blog:

Benefits of Water Therapy

Uddiyana Bandha: Uddiyana Bandha (flying upward) is a famous hatha yoga detoxification technique, which you have probably seen in action if you have ever either seen a yogi in action or attended a hath yoga class. In hatha yoga there are around 80 main asanas or postures. Uddiyana bandha is a subset of this known as bandha (which means hold) and it is seen as a purification technique, which usually takes place in the morning, but actually it can be practiced at any time. In essence uddiyana Bandha is a detox exercise, whereby you suck your navel in towards your backbone while sucking your diaphragm upward (thus named flying upward). The idea is that by sucking in and up, that the intestines will get a nice massage. Actually it's a really good and simple idea, as our intestines tend to get worked hard but they rarely get rest and never get any sort of massage.

Uddiyana bandha is a sort of the grown up version of rubbing a young child's tummy. Why do young kids like this so much? They like it because the gentle rubbing actually relaxes the intestines. With uddiyana bandha, by sucking in and up the intestines suddenly get flushed with blood which takes away toxins, while putting oxygen and nutrients into the gut. Also it relaxes both either stomach wall and the intestinal wall.

Overall uddiyana bandha has the following benefits:

- Better digestion
- Detox of the gastrointestinal system
- Blood purification
- Adrenal glands become more effective
- Improves liver performance
- Improves performance of the pancreas
- Improves blood circulation
- Increases flow of subtle energy through the body

Uddiyana bandha is a simple and effective way of taking toxins out of the gut, while strengthening the walls of the stomach and intestines, as they tone up in the process.

The traditional way to perform uddiyana bandha, is to stand while holding your hands on your thighs; breathe out and then suck in your stomach and then repeat this process several times. This can make many people feel breathless, so another variation on this is to breathe out and then suck in the abdomen once and then out, then breathe in and then out again. This is a slower way to perform uddiyanaa bandha, but I do see benefits of both approaches.

The traditional approach of doing many repetitions in a short burst of time flushes the intestines with blood, but often it does not have much of an effect on subtle energy. The slower approach works better, both for people who have a less well toned abdomen and also for those who are seeking to move subtle healing energies around the body. As a correctly performed uddiyana bandha will definitely lock both the anus and the epiglottis, which holds energy whiten the body.

To achieve this, when in position try when you breath out, to suck into the stomach and feel the epiglottis closing, at the same time try to suck in the anus. From an energetic point of view, this will do you a lot of good, but it has to be performed slowly.

Another variation is to perform uddiyana bandha on all fours. The advantage with this variation is twofold. Firstly it's far easier for people who are overweight, as it is difficult to pull in a big belly. Secondly, it is far easier to pull in the anus and close the epiglottis, just creating a sort of energetic vacuum or lock, which keeps the subtle energy currents inside the body, thus recharging it from the inside.

Uddiyana bandha is a great exercise, but it tends to be performed in a very flashy manner by many hatha yogis who like to show off their abdominal muscle control, while this looks impressive it does not help us in anyway, as we have to rely on our abdominal muscles and not theirs!

That's why I prefer the sitting on all fours method and also taking a more slow approach.

Another even easier variation is to lie on your back and breathe in while expanding your belly. Then breath out and suck in your navel, as if it were intended on making it meet your backbone. This gentle sucking in, will massage the intestines and it's very easy to perform.

The thing to remember about uddiyana bandha, is not to get either excited or put off by watching people in yoga classes or on You Tube, when they perform this exercise, possibly very quickly. The key to making uddiyana bandha work for you is to work at your own pace, concentrate on proper execution and take your time. Also you can increase your amount of reputations over time. Atypically do 10 reps, which is one round, then take a break for a few seconds and then repeat another round and then yet another round. Over time this number can of course increase, but no force should be used.

For more detailed information on uddiyana bandha and a video about it, look here to see my blog article on it:

Healbodymindandspirit.com/How to perform Uddiyana Bandha

A Note on Purification: You might have noticed by now that I am making a big deal about purification and this is simply because when we have gastrointestinal imbalances, toxins build up in the body and the first step in rebalancing everything is to detox the body. Supplements like wheatgrass and Aloe Vera will help, water therapy will help and so too will green tea and uddiyana banda. But one thing which we have to be careful about is detox withdrawal symptoms.

Detox symptoms includes:

- Stomach irritation
- Flatulence
- Diarrhea
- Aches and pains
- Lower back ache
- Flu like symptoms
- Headache
- Dizziness
- Vague feeling in the head
- Irritation
- Anxiety
- Anger

- Depression

I know all of this sounds terrible, but the reason for such symptoms is that as the toxins leave the body, they produce side effects on the way out. Don't give up on the detox, but continue onwards as the symptoms will pass away, in a week or two. Also if the effects are too strong then slow down your pace of change. The emphasize here is sustainable change, as there's no point in being a boy scout for a month and then rebounding back into old habits again!

Realistically speaking it's going to take several months to get the gut back into balance anyway, so take it step by step!

Also think about the many benefits of detox which includes:

- Removal of bodily toxins
- Liver cleansing
- Reduction of inflammation
- Weight Loss
- Increased mental clarity
- Enhanced mood
- Improved self confidence
- Improved sense of well-being
- Improved skin
- More youthful appearance

These are just some of the positive effects of detox. But most people fail to make the restoration of gut health, which they deserve, simply because they feel so bad during the detox process that they give up before the toxins clear out.

Remember, there is a finite amount of toxins and once they clear out, you will feel a lot better in every area of your life, so stick to it.

For more information on handling detox seem toms take a look at this article on my blog here

How to Handle the Effects of Detox

Final Thoughts on Gut Health Rebalancing

Wrapping things up then, we begin with detox and then we move onto rebalancing and rebuilding. How best to do this will depend upon your individual needs. Some people need more rebalancing whilst others require more rebuilding. For example, if you have stomach ulcers rebuilding will definitely be required, whereas if you suffer from food sensitivity, then the focus will be more about rebalancing.

The charts above are a good starting point, but ultimately trial and error is the best way forward, once you understand the general principles of detox rebalance and rebuild. You can heal your gut, but to do so effectively will require patience and forbearance on your part.

The good news about gut health, is that unless you have serious physiological damage to the gut, chances are that gut damage can largely be reversed, to the degree that either you will make a complete recovery or at the very least you will have far better gut health than had prior to been obtained!

Finally remember that everyone is different and that the gut is a large part of the body, going from the mouth done through the stomach, intestines and out through the anus. So while the intention behind this book has been to provide a framework which will help you in the process , the only way to really make good progress is to follow the broad outlines, the general fundamental principles, but trial and error and perseverance are required, in order to heal your gut!

Appendix – 28 Day Gut Restoration Program

There are two messages which I wanted to make while writing this book. Firstly I wanted to get the point across that gut health issues can be cured or greatly improved, but it takes detox, rebalancing, and rebuilding. The second message which I wanted to get across is that every person is different and different approaches have to be taken. Even when similar symptoms are displayed the approach required to bring about cure can differ. So the guiding principles (detox, rebalance, rebuild) are universal, whereas the application of these principles is always individual.

With this in mind I have recommended a self-experimental approach and as a rule of thumb I don't like cookie cutter programs. However, I also know that it can be difficult to make a good start of rehabbing our gut imbalances, and a good start goes a long way towards long-term maintenance. While not ideal for everybody, if you want to have a go at making a big splash with, your gut healing program, then try out this protocol. So with this in mind what follows is a 28 day gut restoration program. It's slightly cookie cutter in its approach and there is a certain amount of sacrifice involved also. But the basic idea is to give your body a break from toxic foods and really give it a good chance to rebalance itself. Also before outlining the steps, I suggest that you keep a journal and note down each day how it is going for you and make changes accordingly as everyone is different.

Food preliminaries

Eat	Don't Eat
Vegetables	Most Dairy Products
Fresh and frozen berries	Gluten products
Lentils	Processed sugar
Quinoa	
Grass-fed meats	Alcohol
Organic eggs	Beverages (regular tea, coffee, all caffeine products)
Fermented foods (Kinchi and sauerkraut)	Rice
Nuts	Beans
Seeds	Soy
Sprouts	Corn
Avocado	Potatoes and Yams
Olive Oil/Coconut Oil	Most Fruits

Ok, I know it's very restrictive, but the idea here is to give your gut a break for a few weeks while rebalancing, so try and stick with it as best you can. As we can see pretty much cereals, breads and even potatoes are of the radar. Pretty much this diet is a meat and veg diet, for most people, and for vegetarians it's a veg and more veg diet. For vegetarian feel free to make very big salads with lots of olive oil or balsamic vinegar as a dressing. Don't worry about the calories, in the oils, as you have to get calories from somewhere, otherwise you will waste away!

For meat eaters this is mainly a high protein diet/moderate fat/very low carbohydrate diet. For vegetarians it is a low protein/ high fat/very low carbohydrate diet. So it's a little extreme but do what you can to maintain it for the 28 days. If you start going potty or find yourself becoming very weak and drawn, then add some foods and beverages back into the mix which you find helpful. Naturally there will be a detoxing withdrawal period of around 2 weeks, where you might not feel all that good. Feeling weak, slightly nauseous, frequent bowel movements and headache are very common symptoms. Also bear in mind that the sudden extraction of carbohydrates, from the diet, will also make you feel a lot weaker after a few days, although by the end of the first week you should be feeling alright again. Also for diabetics keep an eye on your blood sugar levels. By the end of this diet your blood sugars may well have improved, but the lack of carbohydrates might make you a little more prone to hypoglycaemia.

Also in particular for vegetarians the diet can be even more daunting. Carbohydrates and proteins result in an insulin spike but fats don't. So changing to a low protein, high fat diet will make blood sugars tend towards the low level which is good, but they could easily go to low. So make sure, if your diabetic, to have a stash of glucose (such as a glucose sweet or drink) handy, especially for the first few days. If you keep on becoming hypoglycaemic, then make a point of drinking some glucose everyday, so as to maintain the balance.

On a more positive note, this 28 diet will very likely result in weight loss and particularly diabetics will see a good amount of weight loss, as the problem with weight loss and diabetics is that they have uneven insulin levels. When we eat carbohydrates and proteins, our insulin goes high and so insulin is a fat storage hormone. When we starve, our insulin goes low and our human growth hormone (HGH) goes high instead, which is a fat burning hormone. So eating a very low carb diet will reduce insulin levels and increase HGH levels. For the diabetics this diet is fairly low protein, more so than the meat eater version, which will increase HGH even more and reduce insulin even more, so fat loss should certainly take place.

Three meals a Day

The detox program is built up around three meals a day. If you wish to reduce or increase meal numbers please do so, as everyone is different and while some people like to eat only one or two meals a day, others feel bad if they eat less than five or six meals a day.

The important thing is it maintain nutritional intake in a regular way. You might like to eat erratically, but your body likes to eat regularly. Also there are too extremes to avoid. One extreme is gluttony, whereby a person eats and eats and eats and overwhelms their system, and the other is whereby a person hardly eats. Hardly eating will weaken your system and over eating will overwhelm your system. As a rule of thumb both approaches should be avoided!

From the point of view of detoxing we are going to approach the three meals as follows:

Detox Meal
Micronutrient Meal
Macronutrient Meal

Detox Meal: The detox meal is a juice or smoothie and the idea here is to drink the juice or smoothie instead of eating a regular meal. The herbs inside the juice or smoothie, will remove the toxins and also a liquid meal puts very little stress on the gut. Also from the point of view of satiation the detox meal is big, as in about 1 liter or 1.5 pints of juice or smoothie. Also the sheer volume of juice or smoothie means that you're receiving more of a detox!

The Micronutrient Meal: There are two main meals to the detox and both contain micro and macronutrients, as in macronutrients are the carbohydrates, proteins and fats and the micronutrients are the vitamins and minerals etc. However, the micronutrient meal simply means that this meal is focused more upon providing micro nutrients rather than macronutrients.

The micronutrient meal consists of a large salad, made up of mixed vegetables and with the addition of olive oil and or balsamic vinegar for taste and also for calories. The idea here is to fill your body with micronutrients to help the rebuilding process. For people who feel the need for more protein, some protein can be added, but don't go to town on it, as we are trying to detox the gut! If you eat a big green salad everyday, your intake of fibre will be very high and this should help to move toxins from your bowels.

The Macronutrient Meal: This is the main meal of the day, where you eat most of your proteins and carbohydrates, it's also the most calorie dense, meal of the day. The idea behind having just one such meal a day, is to provide sufficient calories and macronutrients while also leaving the gut a chance at self-healing, because one meal is liquid and the other is a salad , so only one is a meal of heavy solids!

Finally, I have labelled the meals as detox, micronutrient and macronutrient, but notice that I didn't mention breakfast lunch or dinner. Whereas most cookie cutter programs believe in setting out everything in stone, I don't believe in taking this approach, as some people need a heavy breakfast and very little food at night, whereas another person only eats at night and yet another person has an average breakfast and a big lunch, with no food at night, for example. So rather than me telling you how to eat and in the process forcing you to eat, in a way which is unnatural for you, then this will not do you good.

Rather in this program we are focused upon one third of food intake being liquid, one third salad and one third full- blown meal. If you stick to these three portion per day, it doesn't matter when you eat your juice or your main meal, for example, so long as you do eat them and also you can go for 2, 3 meals or even 5 or 6 meals a day, so long as it is split accordingly. For example, a person who only wants to eat 2 meals a day could skip the juice/smoothie meal and go for a main meal and a very big salad as the other meal, for instance. While a person who like to eat say 6 times a day could go for 3 juice/smoothie meals and then a salad meal, a homemade meal and a main meal for the final one.

I'm leaving all these options open for everyone is different. A person who is 4 foot tall and weighs 80lbs, is probably going to eat less than someone who is 6 foot five and who weights 300lbs, so how can they be treated the same!

Also one person weighing 180 pounds only needs 2500 calories a day, whereas another person, who weighs in at 180 needs 5000 calories a day!

So just remember everything in this gut restoration program is a guide and is not set in stone. Try and avoid the wrong foods, try and split your food intake into one third liquid, one third salad and one third heavy solid and keep it up for a few weeks and good results shall come!

Detox Shakes and Juices

What follows are 3 shakes and 3 juices. Make a point of taking one each day over the 28 day gut restoration period

Juices

Apples/Oranges & Carrots

Ingredients:

- 2 medium apples
- 2 oranges
- 14 medium sized carrots

Procedure:

1. Peel and chop the fruit and vegetables.
2. Mix all together in a blender.
3. Add 500 ml of water and blend for 1 to 1.5 minutes.

4. Filter using a filter and a large spoon so as to squeeze out the juice.
5. Then take the juice and drink or place in the refrigerator for later.

Benefits:

- Apples are high in insoluble fibre. Because fibre can't be absorbed by the body it has to be excreted and it will help the digestion process while doing this. Also it has pectin, an enzyme which helps to break down food.
- The acids in orange juice help the digestion process.
- Carrots help to cleanse the liver and also stimulate bile production, which is good for digestion. Carrots also boost energy levels and enhance the taste.

Basil, Carrots, lemon & Peaches

Ingredients:

- 3 basil leaves
- 14 carrots
- 1 lemon
- 5 medium sized peaches

Procedure:

1. Peel and chop the fruit and vegetables.
2. Mix all together in a blender.
3. Add 500 ml of water and blend for 1 to 1.5 minutes.

4. Filter using a filter and a large spoon so as to squeeze out the juice.
5. Then take the juice and drink or place in the refrigerator for later.

Benefits:

- Basil helps to improve the digestion process.
- Carrots help to cleanse the liver and also stimulate bile production, which is good for digestion. Carrots also boost energy levels and enhance the taste.
- Lemon juice boosts the digestive process.
- Peaches boost the digestive process, and they also taste really good!

Apples, Lime & Strawberries

Ingredients:

- 2 apples
- One half of a lime
- 3 cups of strawberries

Procedure:

1. Peel and chop the fruit. Mix all together in a blender.
2. Add 500 ml of water and add sugar if you want a sweeter taste.

3. Blend for 1 to 1.5 minutes.
4. Filter using a filter and a large spoon so as to squeeze out the juice.
5. Then take the juice and drink or place in the refrigerator for later.

Benefits:

- Apples are high in insoluble fibre. Because fibre can't be absorbed by the body it has to be excreted and it will help the digestion process while doing this. Also it has pectin, an enzyme which helps to break down food.
- Limes boost digestion.
- Strawberries reduce inflammation of the stomach lining thus relieving gastritis.

Smoothies

Banana Relief

Ingredients:

- 3 bananas
- 2 avocados
- 1 cup of aloe Vera gel or liquid
- 2tbsp's of honey
- 1 cup of ice cubes and 300ml of cold water or 500ml of cold milk or 500ml of natural yoghurt

Procedure:

1. Place the fruit and aloe Vera oil into a blender.
2. Blend until smooth.
3. Add some extra natural yoghurt in if you want to make it more liquid.
4. Add sugar or honey if you want to make sweeter.

Benefits:

Bananas: Contain pectin, which helps with bowel movements. Often stomach aches result from blocked intestines which results in the intestines becoming bigger, which then presses (painfully) against the stomach.

Avocados: Reduce inflammation in the stomach lining.

Aloe Vera: Improves digestive functioning thus relieving stomach ache.

Honey: Reduces inflammation of the oesophagus and stomach lining and also it has a soothing effect which helps both with stomach ache and with acid reflux.

Papaya Yoghurt Twist

Ingredients:

- 1 papaya
- 1 knob of ginger
- 3 tbsp. of honey
- 1 cup of ice cubes and 300ml of cold water or 500ml of cold milk or 500ml of natural yoghurt

Procedure:

1. Place the fruit, yoghurt, ginger and cold water/milk/natural yoghurt into a blender.
2. Blend until smooth.
3. Add some extra natural yoghurt in if you want to make it more liquid.

4.   Add sugar or honey if you want to make sweeter.

Benefits:

Papaya: Helps to settle the stomach

Ginger: Improves the digestive system and also helps out with nausea.

Natural Yoghurt: Is a great probiotic and helps to fill the stomach with friendly bacteria, which aid in digestion. Natural yoghurt is also a base and helps to reduce acidity in the stomach.

Honey: Reduces inflammation of the oesophagus and stomach lining and also it has a soothing effect which helps both with stomach ache and with acid reflux.

Strawberries/Peaches and Natural Yoghurt

Ingredients:

- 3 cups of strawberries
- 5 medium sized peaches
- 1000ml of natural yoghurt

Procedure:

1. Place the fruit and natural yoghurt into a blender.
2. Blend until smooth.
3. Add some extra natural yoghurt or milk in if you want to make it more liquid.
4. Add sugar or honey if you want to make sweeter.

Benefits:

Strawberries: Reduce inflammation of the stomach lining thus relieving gastritis,

Peaches: Boost the digestive process, and they also taste really good!

Honey: Reduces inflammation of the oesophagus and stomach lining and also it has a soothing effect which helps both with stomach ache and with acid reflux.

Micronutrient Meal

The idea behind the macronutrient meal, is to have a meal which is high in vitamins and minerals. With that in mind the micronutrient meal is a big salad. The salads mentioned below are purely vegetarian, but you can add in meat or fish if you like, but do try to keep to light meats or fishes, such as simple chicken breast, turkey breast, salmon or tuna for example. Remember we are trying to ease the burden on our gut, so if you add meat or fish, just add enough to add in some protein and taste, but don't go overboard!

Basic Healthy Salad

Ingredients:
- A handful of kale
- One medium red cabbage/ or one medium sized head of lettuce
- 6 carrots
- 2 medium sized beetroot
- 2 large red peppers
- 2 large yellow peppers
- ½ cup of raw sunflower seeds
- ½ cup of fennel
- ½ cup of sprouted mung beans
- 4 medium sized tomatoes

Dressing:
- ¼ cup of balsamic vinegar
- 2 tablespoons of olive oil
- 1 tsp. of chopped raw garlic

- 1 tsp. of Dijon mustard
- Medium lemon juiced
- ¼ tsp. of salt
- 14/tsp. of pepper

Directions:

The mung beans require a little bit of preparation. Other than that simply chop everything in small pieces, and then add in the various dressings at the end,

Regarding mung beans, to sprout them do as follows:

1). Wash the beans thoroughly in water
2). Leave the beans in a container overnight, with about an inch of water over them and a cover over the box.
3). Next day strain out the water, rinse and refill the water again, and once more leave overnight.
4). Repeat this process until sprouts have formed out of the mung beans, which should take two or three days. These sprouted moon beans are now very nutritious and tasty too.

Kale and Humus Salad

Ingredients:

- 1 head of kale
- 100grams/4 ounces of mushrooms
- 1 large yellow pepper
- 1 large green pepper
- 2 large onions
- 3 medium sized tomatoes
- ½ cup of walnuts or other nuts which you like

Dressing:

- ½ cup of humus
- 2 cloves of garlic
- 1 tablespoon of parsley
- 1 large lemon juiced or two medium lemons juiced
- 3 tablespoons of olive oil
- Salt and pepper to taste

Directions:

Simply slice the vegetables and fry the mushrooms. Then mix in the mushrooms with the vegetables and then add the dressings to taste, mixing everything as you go.

Quinoa Salad

Ingredients:

- 4 cups of cooked quinoa
- ½ a cup of scallions sliced
- 2 large apples (either of green or red variety)
- 1 cup of cranberries
- ½ a cup of nuts of your choice

Dressing:
- 3 tablespoons of honey
- 2 tablespoons of fresh mint
- 1 medium sized lemon juiced
- ½ a cup of olive oil
- Salt and pepper to taste

Directions:

Quinoa Preparation
1. Rinse the quinoa in water so as to clean of any deposits
2. To cook the quinoa, take one and a half cups of quinoa and add in 3 cups of water and heat.
3. After it boils leave it to simmer for 15 minutes while stirring occasionally.

Other than the quinoa simply slice the vegetables and then mix in the quinoa, adding in the dressing at the end.

Citrus and Seed Salad

Ingredients:

- 1 large head of lettuce
- 1 large grapefruit, 1 large orange and 1 medium sized lemon
- 1 tablespoon of sunflower seeds
- 1 tablespoon of pumpkin seeds
- 1 tablespoon of fennel
- ½ cup of olives
- ½ cup of olive oil
- Salt and pepper to taste

Directions:

Simple slice the citrus fruit and add in the seeds and olive oil and salt and mix up and serve.

Mixed Fruit and Berries Salad

Ingredients:

- 1 cup of kale
- 1 large green pepper and 1 large yellow or red pepper
- 1 cup of cherry tomatoes
- 1 orange

- 1 cup of sliced peaches
- 1 large pear
- 1 medium sized bowl of either green or red grapes (ideally red grapes)
- 1 cup of blueberries
- 1 cup of blackberries
- 1 cup of strawberries

Dressing

- 3 tablespoons of honey
- ½ cup of olive oil
- Salt and pepper to taste

Directions:

Just slice mix and serve!

Mixed Veg Salad

Ingredients:

- A handful of broccoli
- The seeds of one large pomegranate
- ½ a cup of fennel
- 2 avocados
- ½ a cup of nuts of your choice
- 1 large orange
- 1 medium sized lemon squeezed

- ½ a cup of olive oil
- Salt and pepper to taste

Directions:

Steam or boil the broccoli until slightly cooked. Chop and mix the vegetables and fruit. Add everything in together and squeeze in lemon juice and add in olive oil, salt and pepper to taste

Macronutrient Meal

The macronutrient meal is very straightforward, simply take one good source of protein such as grass fed beef or fish, for meat eaters, or lentil, quinoa or sprouts for vegetarians and then add in some vegetables as a side order.

The two main things with the macronutrient meal, is to firstly eat enough proteins and fats (we're not too worried about carbohydrates as healthy fats can substitute for starchy carbs) and secondly to satiate ourselves.

The difficult thing with the macronutrient meal is avoiding starchy carbs, which means that unless you eat lots of vegetables, that it can be a little bit unfilling. So to fill out this meal, either eats lots of vegetables and some gut friendly fruits, such s bananas and apples and avocadoes, or simply eat a larger main portion. So maybe two chicken breasts, for example, or if vegetarian cook 3 cups of quinoa and have a really big but simple meal.

Another nice way to fill out the main meal is to either begin with a soup or to make up a casserole or stew, as the mixture of liquids and solids is more satisfying. Below are two examples of dishes which are filling, while also being good for gut health and free of starchy carbohydrates.

Chicken Casserole

Ingredients:

- Four chicken breast with bones (good for health and tasty)
- Chicken stock cubes
- 4 chopped onions
- A small bowl of mushrooms
- 1 cup of sour cream

Directions:

1. Take two chicken stock cubes and melt into a small saucepan of water.
2. Cook the chicken either via frying, grilling or steaming.
3. Take the chicken and the chicken stock and add in the other vegetables into a baking container and place into a preheated oven. Leave in the oven at 350 degrees Fahrenheit (175 Celsius) and leave for half an hour.

Vegetarian Stew

Ingredients:

- 2 onions peeled
- 2 parsnips
- 4 pieces of celery
- 1 pint of vegetable stock
- 6 tomatoes sliced
- Some chopped parsley
- 1 tablespoon of olive oil

Directions:

1. Heat the olive oil in a large pan along with the onions (onions take longest time to cook)
2. Add in the other vegetables
3. Once they are lightly cooked add in the vegetable stock and leave to simmer for a few minutes
4. Once cooked sprinkle with chopped parsley

Supplementation

For supplementation you can add in wheatgrass and aloe Vera for detoxification. Take aloe Vera with every meal and for the duration of the 28 day program take three glasses of wheatgrass a day. Also try out some water therapy, as this will also help to clear out the toxins from the bowels. As always see how it goes and if you find yourself having endless bowel movements, then reduce the intake of wheatgrass and Aloe Vera accordingly.

Another really useful supplement is L-Glutamine, as it's a great rebuilder as well as been a general tonic.

Other supplements such as Kambucha or ACV, for example, would also be a good idea, but the minimum should be wheatgrass, Aloe Vera and L-Glutamine. Other than this, as always green tea is a great detox option which you might consider adding in.

Summing up the 28 Day Gut Restoration Program

As noted at the beginning of this Appendix I'm not a big fan of cookie cutter programs and this is because everyone is different. For example, some people are full-blown meat eaters, others are vegetarians; some pope have serious food allergies and others have no allergies but they have stomach aches and nausea or possible IBS, for example. So there's no way of creating a perfect program.

Also everyone has different lifestyles, with some people liking to eat many meals whereas others want to eat very infrequently, for example. So we have to ask ourselves, when we are considering a 28 detox program, as to what we want to achieve and how we want to go about achieving it.

This is why it has been created to be very flexible, the idea being to avoid foods which are high in toxins, allergic responses or simply hard to digest, while eating other foods, which aid digestion. The daily juice or smoothie will help the detox as so to will the daily salid and the main meal, the macronutrient meal, should be fulfilling and should give enough calories, so as to help maintain the body.

At the same time everyone is different and so you might want to opt for 4 meals a day or 5 meals a day or 2 meals day. But the thing is to try to avoid the foods which have been listed as not so good and to take on average one third of meals in liquid form (as in vegetable juice or smoothie) one meal as a salad and one normal main meal (but without the starchy carbs and cereals).

If you stay fairly true to this diet you wild definitely have a great detox. Taking 28 days out to avoid starchy carbs and cereals, which are prone to gut sensitivity issues, will greatly help to make an easy time for the intestines. The juices and smoothies will remove a lot of toxins, while putting in a lot of vitamins and mineral, thus helping to restore balance and rebuild the gut. Furthermore the large salad will again help with the detox, rebalance and rebuild. While the main macronutrient meal will help to maintain, strengthen and rebuild the body.

You might also have noticed that I haven't outlined each day and each meal and this is because its two restrictive. Mix and match as you need to while trying to avoid the foods quoted earlier and taking one third of your food intake as vegetable liquid, one third as salad and one third as main meal.

It's a very simple yet very detoxifying meal plan. Although it's not without it challenges, as it's a low carbohydrate diet, which will make the first few days challenging. A sudden drop in carbs will make you feel weak and possibly dizzy and also maybe hungry or having lots of sugar cravings, although it will also aid for quick weight loss.

Also another challenge is the lack of beverages and snacks. We human beings are creatures of habit and apart from obvious hunger pangs; we can also suffer from withdrawal pangs. So a good idea is to have some healthy snacks handy. Nuts, raisins, prunes, currants and other such healthy snacks can be imbibed. Also certain fruits can be taken such as apples, bananas and pears. However, bananas while good for the gut, are slow to digest and can result in too much mucus if many of them are eaten. So try to keep snacking, even healthy snacks, like the fruits mentioned above to a minimum. So there's no point, for example, been on a detox and then eating 10 bananas at one sitting!

Finally stick with it for 28 days or at least until you feel you have had enough of the restriction!

If you do it right certainly a big improvement in symptoms will be noted. But also remember to keep up the maintenance. Slowly include a wide variety of foods, over the period of a few days and adjust accordingly. Don't just go back to eating the way you used to eat, as all the good work which you have achieved, over a period of weeks, can be unravelled within a few days!

Finally, it's not necessary for most people to do this 28 day program. Obviously the 28 day program will kick start your gut restoration, but it's easy to get carried away with the gimmicky idea of healing the gut within 28 days. Even if you stick with the program for 28 days, afterwards maintenance is vitally important and this is the most important part of the gut healing program. Whether or not you try out the 28 day protocol, make a point of working on detoxing, rebalancing and rebuilding and be patient enough to keep it up, over a period of months, in order to produce a long-term improvement in gut health!

Thank You

I hope you have enjoyed this book and found it interesting. These herbs are very powerful and are a simple way to support you through the recovery process. But do remember they are a support so don't simply swap allopathic medications for herbs. Both allopathic and herbal formulations are simply there to assist you while you recover.

If you like this book please leave a review for it:

And for more interesting and helpful information, on every suspect of physical, mental, emotional and spiritual health, please visit my website:

healbodymindandspirit.com

Thanks once again for taking the time out to read this book.

Yours in health

Dermot Farrell

Blood Pressure Book

By

Dermot Farrell

healbodymindandspirit.com

MEDICAL DISCLAIMER

The information in this book is not intended to replace professional medical supervision. High blood pressure is a potentially serious health condition and should be regarded with respect. The information in this book is highly effective and it will definitely reduce the blood pressure of nearly every person who earnestly uses the techniques outlined within. In some cases a cure may take place; however, there is no guarantee that high blood pressure will be complete cured. Prior to reducing or stopping blood pressure medications do consult with a qualified physician.

Copyright © 2016 and beyond Dermot Farrell

All Rights Reserved. No part of this publication may be reproduced in any form or by any means, including scanning, photocopying, or otherwise without prior written permission of the copyright holder.

Disclaimer and Terms of Use: The Author and Publisher has strived to be as accurate and complete as possible in the creation of this book, notwithstanding the fact that he does not warrant or represent at any time that the contents within are accurate due to the rapidly changing nature of the Internet. While all attempts have been made to verify information provided in this publication, the Author and Publisher assumes no responsibility for errors, omissions, or contrary interpretation of the subject matter herein. Any perceived slights of specific persons, peoples, or organizations are unintentional. In practical advice books, like anything else in life, there are no guarantees of income made. This book is not intended for use as a source of legal, business, accounting or financial advice. All readers are advised to seek services of competent professionals in legal, business, accounting, and finance field.

First Printing, 2016

PART ONE – OVERVIEW

Chapter One – Getting a handle on Your High Blood Pressure

High blood pressure is at epidemic proportions across the globe. According to The American Heart Foundation, one in three adult Americans has high blood pressure. According to the WHO (World Health Organisation) high blood pressure is listed in the ten most common cause of death and it is obviously a contributing factor to the top two causes of death, which are Ischemic heart disease and stoke respectively. In total 7.5 million deaths (about 12.8% of all the annual deaths worldwide per annum) 1 are as a direct consequence of high blood pressure!

So if you are presently suffering from high blood pressure, you are suffering from one of the most common ailments on the planet and possibly the most deadly ailment, if you suffer from high blood pressure for an extended period of time. Consequently, it is of the utmost importance, for your health, to tackle your blood pressure issues. Fortunately, there are a great many blood pressure medications available, on the market, which can help to control your blood pressure.

But **CONTROL** is the operative word here, as they do not really help your blood pressure (BP), rather than merely reduce the symptoms of BP, which will save you from developing serious health issues such as high cholesterol, heart and kidney disease. But you still have high blood pressure, and this is a concern, because even if your BP is controlled by drugs it can get out of control from time to time and damage can occur. Also, even though blood pressure medications do a good job, of bringing about some level of control, they cannot replace mother nature, so to some degree as long as you have elevated levels of blood pressure some damage is taking place, at some level, in the body. Finally, the drugs themselves have not only side effects, but also they have long term toxicity which will damage the body.

Blood pressure which is only controlled via medication, will in the long-term (over decades in many cases) result in an increase in medications, as the body adapts to various drugs and the overall health balance of the body worsens. Finally in old age blood pressure will result in many complications which will worsen one's health, precipitate other serious health conditions and eventually shorten ones lifespan!

I say these things, not to frighten but rather to motivate you to take some time and effort to work on improving your blood pressure via natural methods. In some cases blood pressure can be completely eliminated, whilst in others it can be greatly reduced. When medical professionals take blood pressure readings they look at two readings, the systolic and the diastolic. In particular the diastolic is the most important reading as it relates to the blood pressure in the arteries, between the beatings of the heart. It is the most important reading because a high systolic reading (blood pressure via the beating heart) can often be high due to physical exertion, such as exercise or running for a bus, however, it does not represent a big health threat, whereas the diastolic does. Take a look below at the box representing the different levels of blood pressure:

Interpretation	Systolic	Diastolic
Normal	120	80
Pre Hypertensive	121-139	81-89
Stage 1	140	90
Stage 2	160	100
Stage 3	180	110
Stage 4	210	120

Don't worry about the exact figures, here are the important findings. An ideal blood pressure rate would be 120/80, although some doctors recommend an even lower figure of 115/75. But what really matters here is that blood pressure, between 75-80 diastolic is very safe. Blood pressure reading 81-89 diastolic represents a risk of hypertension rather than outright hypertension, it suggest prevention rather than a need for cure. However a diastolic reading which is greater than 90 represents high blood pressure, above 100 represents a serious blood pressure condition and above 110 is seen as hypertensive emergency (meaning needing immediate medical intervention which could include hospitalisation), as for 120 plus, well this is an extreme case and would definitely require immediate hospitalisation, in order to reduce the blood pressure levels.

Is it possible to cure high blood pressure?

The answer to this question depends on the level of BP which you are suffering from. If a patient is borderline hypertensive (140/90), for instance, there is a good chance of complete remission, whereas if a patient suffers from stage 3 hypertension (180/110) and has done so for many years, then they will be less likely to be able to cure their high blood pressure, however, they can definitely greatly reduce it. For example, they might be able to get down to stage 2 (160/100) or perhaps, in some cases, even manage to get back down to the borderline hypertensive state (140/90). In some cases a complete remission may even be possible, but this will only be in rare cases. I am saying this because it is important to have a realistic expectation about the degree of cure.

It's important to realise the power of complementary medicine, but also it is equally important to recognise that (regardless of what you might read on some websites) there is no magic cure-all pill to every human health problem.

There are two equally dangerous assumptions which could hinder your ability to cure yourself (or really improve your BP) of hypertension and they are:

1) There is no cure for hypertension; you just have to eat pills for the rest of your life.
2) There is a magic cure which will complete irradiate your hypertension in less than 30 days!

Both of these myths will hinder you. The first myth, the allopathic myth that blood pressure cannot be improved and that drugs are required for life, is based upon an inability for allopathic medicine to explain how exactly blood pressure takes place and hence they are not sure of how to cure it. They suggest lifestyle changes and if they don't work, then they suggest drugs. Since allopathic medicine tends to presume its superiority over and above all other health systems, it therefor concludes that pills are necessary for life, which of course is patently untrue!

The reverse myth, that allopathy is stupid and that only natural cures work, is equally doomed to failure. If you can completely turn around your hypertension in 30 days, then you really have a very minor case of BP to begin with. The natural methods suggested in this book do work, but they work naturally over time. Yes a great result will take place within 30 days, I can assure you of that, however, and they are not a panacea. In cases of mild BP they will completely irradiate it, quite possible in as little as 30 days, and in cases of more severe hypertension they will radically improve the condition within 30 days, though a cure is not guaranteed.

What I suggest is to take the common sense approach that both allopathic and complementary medicine have their respective uses. Allopathy, for instance, is a great way to control blood pressure while you take other natural measures to cure the root cause of blood pressure, remembering that pills can never do this.

I know that some complementary health practitioners recommend that you throw your pills away on day one as pills are toxic. However, I would never suggest such a crazy thing as these pills are preventing organic damage; rather reduce your blood pressure and then lower down the dosages of blood pressure medications over time, possibly stopping them altogether within a few weeks or months of beginning this program.

Who is Dermot Farrell and why should you listen to his advice

I'm not claiming to be a great healer or an all knowing person, but I did spend three years training in Traditional Chinese Medicine and I do hold a diploma which reflects this. Over my years of study I came to understand hypertension, from a complementary perspective, and rather than condemning the allopathic approach I learned to see how each approach is relevant in its own way. However, complementary health systems see the bigger picture, whereas allopathy only sees the symptoms. Since allopathy cannot comprehend the cause, it is hardly likely that they could advocate the cure! Whereas complementary medicine points towards the cure, allopathy helps maintain a degree of control of the symptoms, which can deter a worsening of the condition until the natural remedies kick into effect.

So back to expectations, I recommend to all of you to take your blood pressure in hand and make a concerted effort to improve it. If you cure it completely then great and even if you only reduce it, it still represents a serious relief to your body, which will spare future symptoms and worsening health conditions.

What follows in each section is a description of tactics which will help to cure your BP. For these tactics do work, however, it is important to be consistent. So rather than trying to incorporate twenty tactics into your life in week one, it makes more sense to import a few tactics per week and increase over time. As a rule of thumb it takes 21 days to reinforce a habit, so think in terms of initiating these changes over a period of a couple moths, rather than going hell for leather on day one and crashing on week two!

Also, for natural remedies to work, it is important to be enthusiastic about them. So rather than feeling like you must systematically follow every tactic proposed herein, rather pick out the tactics which you feel would be interesting or pleasant or really worthwhile. Give them a go for a couple of weeks and then add in other tactics as needed, this way it's an organic approach to lowering your blood pressure.

The thing which you have to avoid is starting today, been really enthusiastic and then seeing no result after say two weeks just dropping it. No don't think this way, rather approach reducing your BP, and improving you overall health, the same way you would approach taking up a new hobby. If you took up guitar playing tomorrow, would you expect brilliance in a month? If you started tennis lessons would you expect to be a competitive tennis player in a week? No of course not, so try making some new changes, every week, and over a period of time work towards improving your overall health and wellbeing. After all If you are now suffering from high blood pressure, I can assure you that it took more than 30 days to initialise, rather it took months possibly years of wrong lifestyle/life stresses etc. to so disrupt your bodies health so as to create the imbalance, which is labelled by allopathic medicine as high blood pressure, and as such at least a few weeks/months will be required to remedy this imbalance!

Don't Drop the Medication

Another important point to remember is that allopathic medication is a very good way to keep blood pressure levels in check. While this is not good in the long term (because of potential side effects) it is a good way to at least prevent immediate damage, to the organs and the cardiovascular system. So rather then drop medications, it is a better idea to keep a record of your blood pressure and as blood pressure levels come down, slowly roll back the medications until a stage is reached whereby you can live healthily without them. Once an average blood pressure reading of around 130/90 is reached and maintained (without medication) then it is safe to do without the medication.

If you are unsure what to do then contact your family physician and ask for their advice. But do remember that many allopathic physicians have been thought that once on blood pressure medication, always on blood pressure medication. So they might be critical of your desire to leave reduce and possible stop taking BP medicines.

There are two extremes here. On the one side are natural health enthusiasts who suggest dropping all pills immediately. However, this is a mistake, particularly with blood pressure medication as to do without them until normal levels have returned, is asking for cardiovascular and systematic organ damage, and of course the possibility of a sudden acute and maybe potentially lethal cardiovascular event , such as a stroke or a heart attack. So I strongly advise you to keep on your meds!

On the other hand we have old styled doctors, who believe that BP is incurable and this opinion comes from ignorance regarding the actual causes of BP. For many people a cure is possible while for others a great alleviation of symptoms and reduction in BP levels is doable. If your doctor flatly denies a possibility of life without blood pressure medication, while your blood pressure readings are in the lower end of range, then change your doctor. It is possible to go without blood pressure medication in many cases. However, as long as you are taking medications multiple times a day, this will never occur because your body gets used to been on medication and actually ends up requiring medication, just to maintain a normalise level of blood pressure.

Hence the only safe and constructive way to reduce blood pressure medicine, is first of all to improve your blood pressure and then slowly reduce over time, do it naturally, systematically, slowly and carefully!

The Importance of Measurement and Record keeping

One more final consideration is measurement and record keeping. Measurement means taking blood pressure readings. I know you will have had your blood pressure tested by a doctor in order to be diagnosed with high blood pressure. But how often will this be, as in once a month, once a quarter, or even once a year?

No it is important for anyone, with high blood pressure, to test at least once a month and during transition periods (as in trying out new medications, hypertensive crises, trying out natural cures etc.) to be far more frequent as in daily, possibly as much as three times a day, in some cases. Now you can hardly achieve this if you have to run down to your doctor every time. Rather take the time out to invest in a blood pressure testing kit. The old manual way using a mercury sphygmomanometer and Stethoscope is the most accurate way to do this, although it's not for everyone, as it is awkward to do and you need someone to demonstrate it in the first place.

An easier solution is an electronic kit, which is really easy to use, but they tend to become inaccurate over time, so if you choose one of those handy self-testing kits do cross check them against your doctor's manual kit at least once a year. Pricing for a good brand name blood pressure tester is around $50, but its well worth the investment as it allows you to check your blood pressure levels very frequently and from the comfort of your own home!

So record keeping, record keeping entails keeping a daily record with your blood pressure testing kit from the first day you start this program. Keep an excel sheet, or simply note it down in a notebook, but do test daily and see how it is improving over say a week, a month a quarter, this way you have objective proof of how you're doing. Also, you can dazzle your doctor on your next visit with your new found knowledge of blood pressure rates as well as a concrete record of how natural remedies have helped reduce your BP. Doctors need all the evidence they can get, as they tend to hear a lot of hearsay. When we give them good facts they tend to become more open to suggesting natural solutions to their patients!

Chapter Two - High Blood Pressure Potential Dangers and Causes

In this section we will take a deeper look at the theoretical side of the causes of high blood pressure. If you dislike reading about theory then just skip ahead to the next chapters, which are all practical in nature.

Potential Dangers

The causes of high blood pressure are manifold, and often it is difficult to find the exact root cause. From an allopathic standpoint, blood pressure arises out of a difficulty in pumping enough blood, around the body, in order to service the various organs and cells in an effective manner. If the body struggles to pump enough blood, around the cardiovascular system, then the heart has no other option but to push more strongly, in an effort to feed the cells of the body and it is this increased pressure which is commonly known as high blood pressure.

The purpose of blood pressure is so that the various cells and organs of the body receive the blood, which is required, in order to both provide nutrients on the one hand and also to take away toxins on the other. If for some reason a particular part of the body fails to receive enough blood, the cells will die, which is referred to as ischemia. So the initial effects of high blood pressure are to serve the cells and organs so as to maintain health. This is good in the short -term, however, in the long-term problems do arrive.

Basically the increased blood pressure puts a lot of strain on the heart which results in left ventricular hypertrophy (LVH) which in and of itself is not harmful (unless it became excessively hypertrophic). Left ventricular hypotrophy, in layman's terms, can be described as the enlarging of the left ventricle (heart chamber), whereby the heart muscle becomes bigger due to the increased workload required to pump the blood. So just like your arm muscles will become bigger, if you lift heavy weights so too will your heart grow bigger too.

So what is the downside of a bigger heart?

The problem with a bigger heart is that it puts more pressure on the arteries and also on the kidneys. For example, over a long period of time some kidney damage can ensue from the increased blood pressure. Also in tandem, once kidney function becomes seriously impaired it can result in a backup of fluids into the heart, which results in a serious and presently incurable condition which is known as congestive heart failure (CHF), which is a degenerative and potentially lethal heart condition.

Another effect of the increased pressure in the blood flow is hardening of the arteries. Everyone has heard of cholesterol, so what exactly is the effect of cholesterol on the body?

Cholesterol is a complex chemical, which depending upon the type of cholesterol can either be good or bad. The bad cholesterol results in the build-up of plaque deposits, much like the plaque which we see on our teeth. Now this plaque can build up in the arteries, and over time both harden the arteries so that they become less flexible, and also they can reduce the inner diameter of the arteries, which in turn makes it more difficult for the blood to flow.

One of the possible causes of high blood pressure can be as a result of the hardening and narrowing of the arteries over time. Bu also an effect of high blood pressure is that the plaque is blasted, under pressure, onto the walls of the arteries thus making the plaque build-up process faster and more destructive. It must be remembered that plaque build-up is common and in mild cases it will probably not cause any bad effects, but severe plaque build-up is really dangerous and can result in such things as either embolisms (otherwise known as blood clots) or ruptures in the arterial walls.

Blood clots often result from a narrowing of the arteries which can be really dangerous, because they are lumps of blood which grow at areas of resistance in the arteries, whereby the arteries have narrowed and some of the blood has been stopped from getting through. So over time it develops into a clot and this clot, will eventually go wither block this artery completely or it will go through the artery. Once through the artery it can result in damage anywhere, which are usually the heart, lungs or brain. A block in any of these organs can result in either severe acute ill health or possibly even instantaneous death! Although in some cases the clot will break down and become harmless, but it's very risky and we should do our best to avoid the growth of blood clots!

As for a rupture it can cause a sudden blowout, such as a haemorrhage (blood leak) in the brain which can cause a stroke or an arterial rupture near the heart, such as a burst aortic artery, which usually results in immediate death!

These are appalling consequences and of course they are at the extreme end, on the lower end we see such things as eye damage due to narrowing of the veins to the eyes, erectile dysfunction, painful intercourse, varicose and spider veins and brittle bones.

Another dangerous consequence of high blood pressure is the implicit damage which is taking place within the body in the form of increased vascular damage which leads onto other health conditions. Looking at the top two causes of death, which are ischemic heart disease and stroke, blood pressure has a strong influence on the development of these ailments.

While it is important to realise the potentially high risk to health, which high blood pressure possesses, it is equally important to realise that high blood pressure is not a disease rather it is a condition. While we might suffer from high BP, ultimately it is a bodily imbalance rather than a disease in and of itself. However, if left unchecked, over a period of months and years, other degenerative diseases will come about as a result if it.

Allopathic Causes

From an allopathic point of view high blood pressure is a consequence of various bodily imbalances such as:

- Poor lifestyle choices
- Obesity
- High fat diet
- Sleep Apnoea
- Age
- Genetics

Poor lifestyle choices really cover all of the first three major causes of hypertension, which include obesity and diet. Typically a person who is physically inactive will have poor circulation. Largely as a consequence of our modern sedentary lifestyle, many people are suffering the effects of poor circulation, and an extreme example of this is Deep Vein Thrombosis (DVT), where a person sits still for a very long period of time and ends up suffering a possibly fatal thrombosis. If you have been on a long haul flight lately, you will probably have read about physical exercises in the 'inflight magazine', well these exercises and advice written therein are aimed at reducing the risk of Deep Vein Thrombosis.

Sedentary lifestyle also inclines many people towards obesity, which further restricts circulation. Poor health choices involving processed foods result in a high fat, high sodium diet which also ravages the cardiovascular system and results in a narrowing of the arteries, which produces high blood pressure.

Other potential causes include sleep apnoea, where a person (usually an obese) person stops breathing, for a few seconds while sleeping, which places the heart under pressure and which can result in elevated blood pressure elves. The other factors then are age related cardiovascular degeneration and of course genetic predisposition.

Please note that apart from age and genetics, high blood pressure is largely caused by an inactive lifestyle, poor appetite and also stress while not directly contributing to the development of high blood pressure, certainly stress combined with fatigue aggravate the condition.

Traditional Chinese Medicine Causes

Traditional Chinese Medicine also provides an interesting insight into the causes of elevated blood pressure. Traditional Chinese Medicine (TCM) outlines the body as consisting of various meridians (energetic channels) which link the bodily organs (zang fu). Depending upon various factors, these channels can either suffer from deficient, stagnant or excessive flow of qi energy. Qi been a form of energy which constitutes everything in the known universe. For example, the chair which you are sitting on is a condensed form of Qi, whist the air which you are breathing is a fairly dilute version of Qi energy. Furthermore we have ying and yang energy. Yang is active and masculine, whereas ying is passive and feminine.

We do not have to understand any of these concepts in detail, as it would take thousands of pages to do all of them justice, but we can learn something by looking at some of the causes of high blood pressure from a TCM perspective.

In TCM the organs are entitled 'zang Fu' and they have a major effect upon Qi energy. The zang organs are ying (nurturing in nature) and these include the heart, liver, spleen, kidneys and lungs. The fu refers to the yang organs, which are the small intestine, large intestine, gall bladder, urinary bladder, stomach and triple burner (sanjiao) channels.

To clarify, these organs do not refer to actual physical organs, rather they are labels which were given many thousands of years ago, by ancient TCM practitioners, in an effort to understand the human body. In some cases there is a correlation between the zang fu and their physical counterparts, but most of the time they refer to energies within the human body.

Each zang fu controls a particular function or activity of the human body and when the Qi energy goes out of balance, within that organ (remember deficient, stagnant or excess), physical symptoms will begin to arise.

How does this relate back to hypertension?

Well specific organs when out of balance have a big effect upon the blood pressure of the body. Let's take a look at the following organs:

Liver:

Forget about your physical liver, rather think in terms of energy. This is what the liver zang is all about, the liver zang is required to move energy smoothly around the body. Now the problem with liver energy is that frequently, when we are angry but have no way to creatively venting our anger, this results in an imbalance in the liver, whereby the frustration builds up over time and depending upon individual genetics and the lifestyle, of the person, the liver may become either deficient, stagnate or excessive. There are many possibly patterns here and to form an exact diagnosis requires regular visits to a TCM practitioner, but for now just think in terms of a bottling up of energy, which in turn results in either a deficiency of energy, required to move the blood, or an excess of energy which is uncontrolled. In each case high blood pressure will ensue.

Kidney:

From a TCM perspective the kidneys help to create yang and ying energy. Deficiency of kidney yang, will result in an imbalance of the heart energy, which in turn produces a pounding of the heart and palpitations. In this case the deficient kidney yang energy, will weaken the hearts ability to pump efficiently, which in turn results in hypertension. Also, in the case of kidney ying deficiency, the kidney in is necessary to sooth the heart, so if the ying becomes deficient, the heart will blaze and an excess condition in the heart will occur which in turn will result in elevated blood pressure levels.

Heart:

The heart energy is necessary for the smooth flow of Qi, which in turn results in balanced blood pressure. When the heart lacks support from the kidney energy, high blood pressure of either a deficient or excessive nature will occur.

Spleen:

The spleen zang is required to regulate water through the human body. One of the conditions which result out of a define of spleen Qi is phlegm (otherwise known as mucus). Phlegm can cause a variety of problems, but from a TCM perspective one of the problems which can result, from phlegm, is a blockage of energy through the body, which in turn impedes the smooth flow of blood, which then forces the blood pressure up in an effort to get the blood to flow more freely.

Take a look at the chart below to see the effect of various organs and how imbalances in them result in a wide variety of symptoms as well as high blood pressure.

Zang Fu/Condition	Symptoms
Liver Fire	Dizziness, distending feeling in the head, headaches near the temples, ringing in the ears, red swollen and sore eyes, bitter taste in the mouth, red flushed face, irritability & possible fits of anger
Liver Yang Rising	Headaches, ringing in the ears, dizziness, head distended feeling, heavy headedness, dryness in mouth and throat, insomnia, vivid dreams, restlessness, irritability, angry,
Liver Wind	Tremor, fever, dizziness, numbness, thirst, flushed face, red eyes, dark urine
Liver Ying Deficiency	Dizziness, blurred vision, dull pain in the ribs, dry mouth and throat, heat in the palms and the soles of the feet
Kidney Yang Deficiency	Lower back dull ache, feeling cold, cold knees, clear colourless urine, frequent nightime urination, water retention (oedema)
Kidney Ying Deficiency	Weak and sore lower back, ringing in the ears, dizziness, sweating, constipation, dry mouth and throat, hot feeling in soles of feet and palms of the hand, spontaneous sweating
Spleen Deficiency - Phlegm	Distinding feeling in head, heaviness of head, chest stuffiness, poor appetite, nausea, insomnia
Heart yang Deficiency	Palpitations, fatigue, shortness of breath on exertion, sweating, discomfort in chest, a sensation of coldness in the hands and limbs, bright pale face
Heart Ying	Anxiety, mental restlessness, fatigue, easily startled, palpitations,

Deficiency	insomnia, dizziness, feel hot and irritated, warm hands and feet, warm chest, dry eyes, dry mouth and throat, thirst

You might well note that the above table lists a huge variety of symptoms and that many symptoms are the same, even though the health imbalances are different. This is because in Traditional Chinese Medicine, the symptom and cause are not directly linked, whereas in allopathic medicine, for instance, there is a tendency to treat the symptom, as if it were a cause. For example, high blood pressure has to be lowered, so the doctor gives a blood pressure lowering drug and some life advice. But that's about it. Why? Because allopathic medicine does not consider blood pressure to be a result of anything other than:

- Poor lifestyle choices
- Obesity
- High fat diet
- Sleep Apnoea
- Age
- Genetics

Whereas, with TCM the causes of high blood pressure are quite varied and include the other symptoms listed above. For example, a patient who has high blood pressure, a lot of mental anxiety, palpitations, insomnia and irritability may well have a heart ying condition, at the root of the blood pressure. Obviously if you understand the root cause of the increased blood procedure, there is a good chance that the condition can be cured or at least featly alleviated!

A word of warning!

We have just taken a very quick overview into TCM medicine and how each organ can energetically affect one's health, in a manner which can result in high blood pressure, alongside a plethora of other health imbalances. However, the above table is not intended to be a conclusive list, far from it. Traditional Chinese Medicine is a vast system, which has endless possible interpretations, which can be made regarding any and all health conditions. So please don't self-diagnose. Even if you take the time out to consult with a TCM practitioner, it is quite likely that it will take several sessions, in order to diagnose your condition, and even then some level of doubt often remains.

Rather I hope that these descriptions will help you to realise that high blood pressure is not a disease, nor is it incurable, nor are its causes nearly as general as you might have been lead to believe. Traditional Chinese Medicine teaches us that the human body is a highly complex organism and that various imbalances can create a variety of symptoms and that one of these symptoms is high BP.

From a TCM perspective, a patient does not suffer from hypertension, rather hypertension is just another symptom of an energetic imbalance!

We could get very technical about the root causes of high blood pressure, from a TCM perspective, but that is not necessary if we want to improve our health.

Rather in order to balance our bodies we need to take some corrective action, this is the main thing.

Where Allopathy meets TCM

Although western allopathic medicine differs widely in its understanding as to the causes of high blood pressure, there is some crossover.

For example, how do the zang fu become unbalanced?

The answer to this question is by life stresses and poor lifestyle choices, which is very similar to the allopathic viewpoint.

Liver: Liver energy will get disturbed by emotional tensions

Kidney: Kidney energy will become unbalanced as a consequence of over work

Spleen: Spleen energy will become unbalanced as a consequence of over work and too much mental tension and worry and a diet consisting of greasy foods.

Heart: Will become unbalanced as a consequence of too much mental tension, anxiety and sadness

So while we see a more detailed outline with TCM, we still see an emerging pattern, that of too much stress, poor diet and lack of exercise.

If we delve a little deeper into TCM theory we come to realise that we have energetic reserves which are known as Qi and essence (essence been the precursor to Qi). Unlike allopathic medicine, in TCM the belief is that each organ has a certain level of energetic reserves and that once depleted a problem will occur. Usually a deficiency will take place either in the yang (active) or ying (passive) energy of a particular yang organ, then this deficiency will set of a chain of events, in this organ, which will result either in a stagnation, deficiency or excess of Qi energy. Like a pack of dominoes, this now dysfunctional energy channel will topple over other channels causing disruption here and there. Finally, according to one's lifestyle and genetic predispositions certain health imbalances will occur. For example, one person might end up suffering from gastric issues, while another person might end up suffering from high blood pressure, simply because the way the energy channels are set up in their body and the lifestyle which they follow.

The good news about this is that we don't have to get hung up on the finer details, rather it is enough to know that we have to recharge all the major organs and energy channels, in order to bring about good health.

Allopathic medicine will recommend lifestyle changes and drugs, but really they do not have a fine detailed comprehension of the root causes of high BP, so they cannot go beyond this. However, by applying some Traditional Chinese Medical principles, we will learn that we can recharge our inner energetic dynamics and in so doing so we can either cure our hypertension completely or at least we can radically reduce it.

In the following sections we will leave theory behind and focus on practical strategies, which are dinged to help either cure or greater alleviate your high blood pressure.

PART TWO – PRACTICAL STRATEGIES

Chapter Three - Lifestyle Changes

The modern sedentary lifestyle goes against two million years of evolution. Up until the industrial revolution, human beings were spending their time either living off the land, initially as gatherers picking whatever fruit or berries or anything that they could find and later as farmers, or as hunters. Think for a minute about this lifestyle; it is a lifestyle of endless physical activity requiring physical fitness and endurance. Also, from a diet point of view, humans had periods of feast and periods of famine. If you successfully hunt down and kill a large animal today, then it's a feast. However, if it's mid-winter and you are out of cereal grains and fruits to eat and hunting is going badly, then you fast for a few days or possibly weeks!

Whichever way you look at it, ancient man was a tough and hardy animal, capable of surviving in tough terrains, in difficult weather conditions and often having to go long periods of time without food and usually having to exercise for at least several house a day.

Modern man, in contrast, is physical inactive and eats far too much. This change started to take place with the advent of the industrial revolution, and with the passing of each decade since the early 1800's human beings have become increasing sedentary, in their lifestyle, to the degree that now a day's most of us are extremely inactive.

Another thing to think about is food. Infant mortality rates have greatly reduced, over the last one hundred years, which is a great thing, however, the massive increase in world population (up from 1.6 billion people in 1900 to 7.3 billion people by 2015) 2 has placed a huge strain on food production.

Consequently, starting in the 1950's, there has been a focus on increasing food production, via artificial fertilisers, as well as an enormous increase in the percentage of processed food. The problems which arise out of this, are foods which are low in bio availability (meaning it is difficult to gain nutrition from them), in the case of crops produced via artificial fertilisers. Also, in the case of processed foods, once again they are often lacking in nutrients, plus they are often filled with chemical preservatives. On top of that most processed foods come with added sugar and salt, which of course is not so good for health.

For example, back in 1900 the average American consumed 112 grams (about a quarter of a pound) 3 of sugar per day, whereas the average American in 2009 consumer 227grams (about half a pound) 3 of sugar per day. So this represents a 100% increase in sugar consumption!

What's so bad about sugar?

Sugar is basically a form of simple carbohydrates, which are good for the fast release of energy. The other type of carbohydrate, complex carbohydrates, releases energy over a longer period of time. Food such as oats, sweet potatoes and brown rice are all slow acting, whereas processed white sugar, bread and corn syrup are examples of fast releasing carbohydrates.

While a small amount of fast acting carbohydrates is good, in that they give one an energetic pick up, too much is a bad thing. The biggest consequence of too many simple carbohydrates, in our diet, is an overloading of the pancreas which has to produce insulin, in order to maintain blood sugar levels. This brings on the onset of diabetes, which in turn often results in obesity plus cardiovascular damage. And of course, obesity will also increase the stress on the heart, as it has to pump blood around a now enlarged body. Finally, obese people usually have an increase of bad cholesterol, which in turn results in plaque build-up in the arteries which of course increase blood pressure.

Sodium is another dangerous food additive. We all like salt, in our food of course, and for commercial food processors salt is a great way of making an otherwise boring food taste better. While some sodium is necessary for health, increased levels of sodium are bad for our heart. In a study on salt consumption in America, it was found that the average American consumed, on average, 3,592mg of sodium per day, which is well above the recommended rate of 2,300mg per day4. Not only that but the study concluded that 90% of Americans consumed too much sodium!

The problem with sodium, is that it encourages water retention in the body. This increased water retention is not just in the cells of our organs, it also is found in the blood. An increase of water, in the blood, makes the blood thicker and consequently it becomes more difficult to up pump this increased volume of blood around the body, which in turn forces the body to increase the blood pressure, in an effort to deliver the blood to all the cells.

The real problem, with sodium and simple carbohydrates, is not that we eat them but rather that they are hidden in our food and often we do not even realise that we are eating them. For example, there is sugar and salt in your bread and your cornflakes. Bread and cornflakes don't taste salty or sugary, yet they are there. Take a quick look around your kitchen. Look at all the canned food and packaged food, on your shelf's and in your refrigerator, and chances are that most of these foods contain salt and sugar. It's hard to believe yet it's true. Obviously we all know that candy bars contain sugar and French fries contain salt, but it is unsettling to think that so many non-sugary non salty tasting foods are full of these unhealthy additives.

Its fine to eat sugar and salt, but it is important that we keep our consumption within limits. Consequently, it is a useful exercise to take a look at the food you eat and become aware of added salt and sugars.

In many cases, simple changes can greatly reduce the sugar and salt levels in your diet!

For example, rock salt is high in potassium so it elevates the sodium effect of processed salt. Just try some rock salt, in your local store, and already you are on your way to decreasing your sodium intake. Another option is to buy low sodium salt, which is good if you cannot find rock salt or if you don't like it.

Probably the easiest way to reduce, hidden sodium and salt, is to reduce your intake of processed food. I know it is difficult, in this day and age to prepare food at home, but where possible try to prepare at least some home cooked food some of the time. As a general rule of thumb, if you make it yourself it's probably good, or at least you will know what went into the food!

Another healthy option, and a practical one in today's busy world, is to locate some healthy restaurants. In every city in the world there are restaurants and café's which specialise in healthy food options. Do your really need those French fries and cheese burgers? Even if you do, there are probably a couple of restaurants, in you city or town, which make relatively healthy home cooked burgers and French fries, rather than the highly processed food items which you will come across in your regular 'greasy spoon' restaurant or fast food outlet.

These are small yet highly effective strategies, which you can take which cost nothing, taste good and will promote a natural reduction in your blood pressure levels, so don't delay start making these simple changes today!

Fat. Fat is the big one. Fat is everywhere in today's typical diet. We eat too much fatty foods, as in French fries and cheeseburgers, pizzas laden with cheese, candy bars etc. According to the American heart Association a person should consume no more than 5% to 6% of their daily calories in saturated fat 6. So for a person on 2000 calories a day this represents no more than 11 to 13 of saturated fat per day, and that's the entire day!

McDonald's Big Mac, for example, contains 8 grams of saturated fat, which is 60% to 70%of an average person's daily allowance. It also contains 1007.4mg of sodium, which is about 50% of one's daily allowance. That's just one burger, what about the fries? What about if you go to Burger King and eat their half pound burger? Get the idea!!!!!....It's really easy to eat too much fat and sodium!

So by eating too much food, we end up becoming over weight, which in turn inclines the body towards developing high blood pressure levels, in order to push the blood around the body. Also, if we eat a diet which is high in sodium, it will increase water retention, thus resulting in increased blood volume and once again higher blood pressure levels. Finally, if we eat a diet which is high in saturated fats, it will incline the body to produce more cholesterol, which in turn will increase the likelihood of developing arterial plaque, which in turn pushes up blood pressure levels, in order to push the blood through narrower arteries!

Probably the single biggest cause of obesity, diabetes and heart disease in our society, today, is overeating. There's absolutely nothing wrong with having a treat. Sugars, sodium and fat are not intrinsically unhealthy, however, in large does they are bad for you. Look at the table below outlining the average quantities of food, consumed by American in the 1970's versus today's figures.

Annual Food in lbs. per Capita	1970-79	2000
Total Meats	138.2	195.2
Fish and Shell Fish	10.9	15.2
Total Fats	53.4	74.5

Total Grain Products	155.4	199.9
Total Caloric Sweeteners	123.7	152.4
Total Fruits and Vegetables	587.5	707.7
All Dairy Products	548	593
Cheese	14.4	29.8
Whole Milk	21.7	8.1
Low Fat Milk	8.1	14.5
Annual Foods by Units		
Eggs	285	250

It's interesting to note that nearly everything has increased, anywhere from 10% to 50%, depending upon the food item. The only items which seem to be coming down in quantity are milk and eggs, and this is obviously because of an increase in consumption of other food in their place.

The reason why eating so much food, is bad for health, lies in the human body's inability to cope with excessive amounts of food, over and above the basal metabolic needs of the body. Put it this way, if a person requires say 2000 calories, in order to maintain their weight, then if they eat on average 2700 calories per day, they will have eaten an extra 21000 calories within 30 days and will definitely be increasing their body fat levels. Presently obesity is at epidemic levels in many countries. Once again if we look at America, for example one third of the adult population are obese[7]. It's very simple math, just eat too much food on a daily basis and you will become fat!

Obesity obviously has an effect on our BP levels, but also it must be noted that when a person eats a lot of food, their overall percentage of sugar, salt and fats ending up increasing too. Even if a person eats reasonably healthy, while been over weight, and only 7% of their food saturated fat, it's 7% of a bigger number. For example, 7% of 2700, for example, is 189 calories, which is 21grams of saturated fat, which is 9 to 11grams above the acceptable level. So the levels recommended, are always based upon a person eating appropriately, for someone with a fairly lean body fat percentage.

Of course, if you're eating junk every day you will raise your blood pressure. But also, even if you eat healthily, if you eat way too much food you will end up consuming too much of the wrong ingredients while at the same time becoming fat.

An example of how this sort of thing can creep up, can be seen when we take a slim person, say a 5 foot 9 inch tall male and he weighs in at a lean 150lbs. He eats more food than his body can handle, and starts gaining weight. In a year he has gained 15lbs, but he doesn't even notice and neither does anyone else. Another year goes by, he gains another 15lbs and people start to notice and comment to him, that he is getting fat. His clothes start to get tight, but he brushes it off and forgets about it. At last another year passes, now he weighs in at a chubby 200lbs and he decides to lose weight. But think about it, is he damaging his body now because he is fat, or was he damaging his body last year when he was chubby, or was he damaging his body the previous year when he was lean? The answer to this questions is that he was damaging his body all along, because even when he was lean he was eating too much food, so he was probably taking in a combination of too much fat, sugar and salt, and so when he develops high blood pressure, it's not suddenly because he is now fat, but rather it so because for three years he has been eating too much of these potentially hazardous foods!

It's a good thing to keep in mind, because some people have high blood pressure and even heart disease, while they are lean. It is possible to have a diet which is very high in saturated fats, for instance, but which is low in calories. In this case you may look nice and lean, but your cholesterol and blood pressure may well be on the rise, don't just judge by outward appearance!

To summarise, this section on healthy eating, do remember that it's not as simple as avoiding the obvious junk foods; it's also about looking out for potential food hazards, in apparently innocent looking food. Also, while obesity can kill, you can also destroy your health while still been slim. Yes it's true that people who are obese are in general more likely to suffer from blood pressure and heart health issues, but if you eat a diet which is high in sodium and saturated fats, then there is a good chance that you will end up with elevated blood pressure, high cholesterol etc. Finally, it's not a difficult thing to eat healthy, rather it's a case of raising our awareness and making informed decisions about our food choices. Often we don't have to go without delicious tasting food, rather we just have to think more carefully about where we eat, what we eat and how much we eat!

Paleo Diet/High Fat/Low Carb/Ketogenic Diets – Cholesterol is Good For You Etc.?????

If you have been reading around the internet, then chances are that you may have read some of this and possibly other confusing material regarding dietary fat, cholesterol and sugar and so on.

In brief summary, the Paleo diet is based upon living like ancient man, eating cruciferous vegetables as the only source of carbs and largely surviving on meat. Other diets, which are similar to this, are known as low carb diets, and ketogenic diets. In the case of the ketogenic diets, the emphasize is upon zero carbs, which force the body into ketosis, whereby the body has to use fats for fuel rather than carbs, as carbohydrates are lacking from this diet.

These low carb diets all claim amazing fat loss possibilities, which is perhaps questionable. But from the respective of elevated blood pressure levels, some of the advocates of low carbs suggest that high carbohydrates are the cause of all modern health problems, and as such things such as high cholesterol and saturated fats are actually either good or at the very least not so bad for us, and rather it's carbohydrates which are causing everything from diabetes to blood pressure to heart disease, and even some people reckon that cancers are caused by high carbs!

Is this the case?

The answer is that we don't really know, as both sides sling mud at each other and hopes it sticks. This leaves us with two distinct possibilities. Either wait for the objective answer to come about, which could take decades of research and debate, or just make a common sense decision about it.

I suggest that you ignore most of this information, for now, and focus upon leading a more balanced life. One factor which rarely emerges from these bombastic debates, between the low carb/high fat lobby (in some cases 50% protein/50% fat) and the established western medical viewpoint(60% carbs/25% protein/15% fat)lobby, is that most scientific research focuses upon an end result rather than taking a look at that test group as a whole.

While there is much differing information, regarding what food is good for you, one thing which appears to be a constant is that people who lead a balanced lifestyle, with a good work life balance, who exercise and eat a good balanced diet tend to fare well in these experiments.

So rather than hopping on the latest diet band wagon, why not try ticking the right boxes first.

Which are?

- Do not over eat
- Try to avoid processed foods
- Try to eat homemade food wherever possible

- Get a good balance of all major food types (so eat fruits, vegetables and good sources of portions)
- Do not eat too much of any one food group
- Exercise regularly
- Don't work too much
- Get a good night's sleep

All of these suggestions are simple and effective, so give these a try before embarking on any weird and wonderful dietary fads.

Also, while I do not want to criticise the low high protein/low carb lobby, as there might be some truth in their assertions, I must advise you that many people have damaged their health by opting for a very high protein/high fat diet. How many grams of protein can the body handle per day without kidney damage ensuing?...it is questionable. Also, while some people advocate a very high fat diet, a lot of people who go on an extremely high fat diet do appear to develop cardiovascular issues, so just be careful.

It seems to me that denying a major food group is probably a bad idea. There are three major food groups, which are proteins, fats and carbohydrates, and they all play their part in human metabolism. To forgo one of these three major groups seems to be to be a risky idea, surely it will result in some imbalance which could cause health problems.

By all means vary the levels of each of these macro nutrients but do try to include them.

Ravaging Effects of Sugar on Our health: One of the arguments of the low carb/high protein/high fat lobby has been the insistence that high sugar levels ravage the body. There may be some truth in this; Dr Richard Johnson, for example, states that high fructose consumption results in an increase in uric acid, which in turn inhibits nitrous oxide, in your arteries, making them less flexible and more prone to high blood pressure8. He goes on to suggest that a uric acid level above 5.5mg per dl increases the risk of hypertension and that glucose mixed with fructose(as in common refined white sugar) increases the absorption of fructose in the body, thus elevating blood pressure levels in the body even more.

This is a fascinating argument, and may prove to be the case, but the debate, for now, continues.

What should we take from this?

Like I said, I think eradicating a primary food group from our diet is probably a bad idea; however, clearly in our modern diet most people are consuming far too many simple carbohydrates (sugars). It would probably be a good idea, for most of us, to either reduce our intake of carbohydrates or at least focus more on complex carbohydrates, such as oats and yams and cruciferous vegetables, such as broccoli and cabbage, as our sources of carbohydrates.

Another promoter of the low carb diet, Gary Taubs (author of 'Good Calories, Bad Calories: Challenging the Conventional Wisdom on Diet, Weight Control and Disease'), proposes that all refined carbohydrates are bad for us. This suggests that not only simple sugars are bad for us, but also oats, and other food sources which consist mainly of complex carbohydrates, are bad for us unless they are unprocessed such as the old slow cooking steel cut oats, for example. If you take a look through a list of processed carbohydrates, I guarantee your disappointment. Very few carbohydrates, even complex ones, fall outside of this list, because in our modern society most foods are processed. Of course, we should try to eat unprocessed foods and this is something which we should all endeavour to do. But it is a difficult task.

Gary Taubs may or may not be right and the low to zero carb lobbies may well have many good points to make, but ultimately we all have to live in the real world, where we have families to run and jobs to keep. So by all means reduce simple carbohydrates and refined carbohydrates, where possible, but accept the fact that it is a tough job to eat perfectly in today's world. I know that for some people eating a diet which is highly unprocessed and organic is an easy thing, whilst for others it is a very difficult thing to do. What we must not do, is simply give up because the task looks too difficult. So take a look at your lifestyle, and see what changes you can do to make your diet healthier. Even if you are not 100% successful, at least some progress will have been made.

Interestingly, when we start to observe our diet and try to make improvements on it, we can see that rubbish foods are everywhere. Just do a little research on food and nutrition, then take a stroll down to your local supermarket and clearly you will see that 75% of all the food stuffs on display are basically rubbish!

It's a tough task to eat a perfect diet in our modern world, especially if you live in a city and your monthly groceries are on a strict budget, but at least try to make improvements. Small improvements will improve not only your blood pressure but many other health factors too!

Finally, the health and diet/fitness market is always coming out with a new diet/improve your health gimmick every year. Right now its low carbs and ketogenic dieting that's all the rage, but do remember that most of these are fads, that just come and go. Try to be reasonable and eat a balanced diet, this is probably the best way to go for most people.

The Importance of Exercise and General Lifestyle Changes

Exercise is an equally important factor in reducing blood pressure issues. Elevated blood pressure levels are a direct consequence of life stress, poor diet and sedentary living. If we cast our minds back to the olden days, when human beings had to hunt and gather for their livelihood, we can see that the human body is designed for exercises. Out of two million years of human evolution, we only see mankind developing a more sedentary lifestyle over the last two hundred and fifty years, and out of that it is the last fifty or so years that sedentary living has really taking root in our society, and the figures back this up. In 1996 only 21% of the US population had high blood pressure versus 31% in 2014!

Simply put our sedentary life combined with a poor diet and stress is literarily killing us!

One of the simplest steps which we can take in order to lower blood pressure is simply to exercise. By exercise I don't mean strenuous weight lifting sessions in the gym or running marathons. Rather just move your body. If your young or even middle aged, and in otherwise good health, then by all means do some strenuous exercise such as the gym, playing squash or tennis or maybe swimming lengths in the pool several times a week. But if you are a little older or maybe obese or your blood pressure is really bad, then please be a little bit more conservative with your efforts.

I have been battling obesity myself for many years and one of the activities which I have emphasized is exercise. But some of my exercise efforts went badly, to say the least. Like the time I decided to climb my staircase (the house which I was living in at the time had a 50 step staircase) fifty times. I did it a few times in a row and then I just started to feell wrecked, so I gave it up. Another time I decided to walk up a mountain (six days a week – bad idea) and once again I felt wrecked. Yet another time I decided to try out skipping (I was weighing in at 265lbs – so not a good idea) and immediately I started having shoulder pain of all things as well as ankle pain.

What's the lesson here?

Well excessive exercise releases cortisol, which is a hormone designed to help in emergency situations. It raises adrenaline levels but it also stresses the body out, thus preventing weight loss and increasing stress and blood pressure!

So exercise yes. Stress yourself out. No!!!

Also, for people who are obese, a lot of exercise involves jumping here and fro, as we see with such activities as skipping and a lot of calisthenics, it's really a bad idea. A 265lb man for example, skipping and jumping around the place is just asking for trouble. Leave the jumping around bit for people who are closer to their ideal weight.

In my case, for example, if I were weighing in at 220lbs then this skipping and jumping would be a good idea, as at 200lbs I would be fairly slim, as I am over six foot tall and have a heavy set build. If I was five foot seven and had a light build then I would have to weigh a lot less before attempting these antics. It all depends upon your physical build, age, level of agility, health problems, aches and pains and so on. What maters here are that exercise should feel doable? If you feel any serious pains and aches then just drop the exercise!

Exercise is a great way to reduce high blood pressure because when we exercise we increase our blood flow, through our bodies. High blood pressure is based upon a foundation of poor circulation; exercise, when done the right way, improves blood circulation. So great, but if you stress yourself out while exercising, then blood pressure will increase, rather than decrease. Also, if your fat and you jump around like a young fit athlete, then chances are you might strain a tendon or a ligament which will put a stop to any exercise activities for a hale!

Rather think in terms of exercise which is DOABLE!

Doable, for one person could mean climbing Mount Everest, whereas for another person it could mean going for a walk around the block! From the point of view of reducing blood pressure, we have to think in terms of regularly moving the body, which in turn will aid the smooth flow of blood.

It's good to get the heart rate up, but not by too much of a degree. The idea, is to gently stimulate your heart and cardiovascular system, so as to improve blood flow. Also, frequency is important; it is better to exercise lightly everyday, than to exercise intensely three days a week. And it is even better to do some light exercise several times a day, from the point of view of blood circulation.

Gently moving the body is good, for blood circulation, and we are designed by nature to be active. Now active doesn't mean performing crazy levels of intense movement, which we see today in many fitness studios. So do try out some exercises, but don't stress yourself out. Be active!

Looking back, at our ancestors, we can see that they were physically active and that also they went through periods of both excessive eating and limited eating, even fasting. When we live closer to how our ancestors live, we are synchronising our bodies with the natural order. Two million years of evolution, has designed humanity to be active and to eat varying amounts of food, with the focus been more on unprocessed foods, with relatively small amounts of carbohydrates, and those carbohydrates been complex and unprocessed in nature. That's how we are made. Two hundred and fifty years, heading in the opposite direction, will not suddenly change our physiology. Perhaps our physiology will change over time, but for now we need to stick close to our natural programming.

We need to live in tune with nature!

Living in tune with nature, does mean been more active and moving away from too many processed foods. But it does not mean jumping onto the next health craze! Beware of health crazes!

Most of the new cool sounding diets, and intense exercise programs, are in fact rehashes of old ideas with gimmicks attached, so as to grab our attention. So next time you see an ad for some new exercise program, cool sounding diet or fat loss thermodynamic herbal tea, just remind yourself that living closer to nature works. You don't have to live a weird unnatural lifestyle, or spend thousands of dollars on questionable supplements, in order to reduce your blood pressure. Rather be active, don't eat too much; fast occasionally; eat mainly unprocessed foods; cut down a little on carbs; try to eat unprocessed carbs where possible; eat junk food less often than you eat healthy foods!

That's it that's all that's needed!

Another factor, which is equally important, is stress. While ancient man suffered from amazing impoverishments, such as famine, fleeing for their lives because of invaders, plagues etc. etc. , on one level their lives were easy in that they didn't have to think too much about a lot of abstract concepts.

For example, I remember in my first job, back in 1989, I got paid every Friday. I received a little brown paper envelope, with my name written on it, and inside it was green folding stuff called cash. That was great, all I had to do was make sure that I still had some of this papery stuff left over until next Friday comes along, when a new brown envelope filled with cash would come along. It was simple living to say the least!

However, now a days most of us are paid electronically into our bank account, on a fixed day every month. We have all sorts of finance going on, from mortgages to car loans, bike loans, holiday loans; we have credit card debts, overdrafts and of course we have health insurance, life insurance, a pension fund and so on. So many complexities, pulling on our purse strings! Kids these days expect better education (meaning mommy and daddy have to save up a fairly big fortune to pay for it!), health insurance, trust funds, pension funds etc. etc.. Also, most of our bills come monthly. For example, TV subscriptions, internet subscriptions, cell phone subscriptions, rent, health insurance etc. And of course, we now have crazily expensive luxury living costs such as smart phone subscriptions charges and various online subscriptions etc., which simply did not exist twenty years ago!

Life has become more complicated and more expensive, a lot more expensive!

For many people, they get paid on say day X each month and two weeks later they are living on fumes! They have no money and are broke, eking out a living for the last two weeks of the month, not because they are poor but rather because so many bills coincide within the week following their pay. Good news is that the rent, phone bill etc. has all been paid, but the bad news is that extra money required for putting gas in our cars and discretionary expenditure is often suddenly lacking, as we move towards our pay day!

Yes our overall finances might be good, but between bills, pensions, trust funds, investment funds etc. we don't have much cash available, in the final week or so of the month, while we are waiting to get paid again. This kind of complex living, creates a funny situation whereby we have money and we are doing well but everything is complex and we end up struggling, sometimes simply for want of better life management, which is difficult to get right in this overly complex word, a world whereby we have a thousand and one things to think about and most of them are about future planning, rather than today!

The simple living, of cash payment once a week and a small few obligations per month, only twenty five years ago, has given way to the investment managed, portfolio based stressed out lifestyle of modern life!

So what are we to do about it?

Well we cannot change the world, or not much anyway, but we can change ourselves; somehow we have to take some time out, in order to get in touch with who are we are. We have to relax and learn to de-stress. Because the world is only going to become more complicated, not less complicated.

So the complexity isn't going anywhere and even attempting to live with nature, as our great grand parents did, is also not really an option. Even old fashions groups, like the Amish people of America, for instance, are finding it increasingly difficult to live like they did in the old days. We can't go back in time, so rather we have to figure out a way of reducing our mental stress and tension, in a world which is rapidly heading towards ever greater levels of complexity!

How to Find Happiness in a Crazy World

So how exactly should we proceed, if we want to lower our blood pressure and maintain our sanity?

Our ancient ancestors were at one with the world, while we are always fighting it dominating it. Humans thirty years ago, were not at one with the world but they had a more easy going life than we have today. No internet, no cell phone, no monthly electronic payments, just cash on a Friday and get on with things until next week.

Maybe trying to get back to the oneness with nature, which ancient man possessed, is now too far from our reach. But what about the relative peace of the person living says thirty years ago? This kind of peacefulness is easier to have than you might think.

Why were people more peaceful thirty years ago, or even twenty years ago, in the pre-internet, pre-cell phone era?

The answer is simple, twenty plus years ago most people were free of the hassle of twenty four hour connectivity. Also, life moved at a slower pace, because everything had to be arranged in advance. Now this isn't saying that life was better, cell phones are great and the internet is great, but where's the peace?

Take Some Time Out

Thankfully we can reclaim some of our old peacefulness by simplifying our lives. The easiest way to do this, is to disconnect from all of these devices, even if only for a few hours. I remember some years ago reading about how the now late actor Larry Hagman of 'Dallas' fame, that he used to make Friday his non speaking day, On Fridays he would make a point of not speaking with anyone. Now that might be a little extreme, but he had a point. Take some time out, switch of your phone (all of them!), disconnect the internet and relax for a few hours. This is such a simple therapy, but it is effective. Ok we can't do it every day, but it is possible to say set aside an evening a week or a Sunday afternoon or whatever and just tell everybody that this is 'me' time and that you're disconnecting for a little while.

The important thing here, is that so many of us get sucked into this crazy endless activity lifestyle because we feel trapped, trapped by endless obligations and yet we don't take out some personal time. Start today and reclaim some time for yourself, it's not been greedy! The people in your life, whom you love, will love you all the more for it because it will help you to become more grounded and peaceful and they will have a better time with you, after the batteries have been recharged.

We're all so quick to recharge our cell phones batteries, our smart phone batteries, our iPad batteries, our laptop batteries, our camera batteries etc., but the one set of batteries which we don't bother recharging are our own!

And recharging our batteries does not necessary mean going to the gym, fitness studio, tennis court, beauty parlour or even for a walk. Let me explain: We have become, as a race, so obsessed by obligations that we drag ourselves everywhere. We drag ourselves to work, we drag ourselves to our parents' house, we drag ourselves to our kids houses, we drag ourselves to the gym, hell we even drag ourselves to the bar or night club. Then when we're all worn out and stressed out with our busy recreational living, we head on into the nearest, every ready, junk food restaurant for a quick refill of garbage dressed as food, which will spike our insulin and make us feel even more stressed out!

The dragging has to stop!

It's not about which recreational activity, which you like to do, but don't let yourself be forced, as it must be genuinely restful. If you go for a walk, relax and don't say to yourself "oh I must complete my forty five minute restful walk!" that's not resting, that's just fulfilling another obligation!

Learn to truly relax and also learn to say no now and again. "No, sorry I can't make it that day", just do it, you owe it to yourself, and to your high blood pressure, to pace yourself. Who said that we have to run around all the time at high speed? We can pace ourselves, why not!

Simplify

Why does life have to be so complex?

Well it doesn't have to be; there is a popular notion going around that we have live in a very complex manner, however, we can decide to change all that. We can simplify our life's, maybe not to the degree of ancient cavemen, but at least to the degree of ordinary people living twenty or thirty years ago on this Earth.

How?

One way we can work towards this, is to complete a LIFE INVENTORY. **A LIFE INVENTORY** is a simple process whereby we overview all major aspects of our life, and we see what needs to stay and what needs to go.

For example, got a gym membership which hasn't be used for six months?

Scrap it!

Paying a TV subscription, every month, but everyone in the house uses either smart phones or the internet to watch TV and movies?

Scrap it!

Do you have three cell phones?

Scrap at least one of them!

Are your wardrobes filled with ten year old cloths' and nick knacks?

Scrap them!

You live twenty five miles from work and have to take two buses to get there?

Move house or move job or buy a car!

Do you feel bad, if you don't visit all three of your best friends, who live very far away from each other, every week?

Tell them you're very busy and stressed out and cut down to visiting one or two friends per week. If they're real friends they'll understand.

So you get the idea, take some time out and go through every aspect of your life, then consider how best to simplify.

While living a simple life is nearly impossible, these days at least, with a little bit of effort and organisation, it is possible to live a far more simple and relaxed lifestyle.

Try this exercise and re-do it at least a couple of times a year and terrific results will come your way!

Love Yourself

Loving ourselves is possibly the hardest thing to do. We think we are loving ourselves, and often times other people will accuse most of us of been in love with ourselves. But this is a different type of love!

Generally speaking, when we talk about someone loving themselves, we tend to suggest that a person has a big ego and who looks after their interests, while ignoring other people's needs and wants. But in reality this is selfishness not love, rather the term self-love is really a bad way of describing selfish behaviour. Selfishness is not love, selfishness is a kind of ignorant self-absorption, but it is certainly not love!

Real love, of oneself, occurs when we learn to accept ourselves as we are, warts and all. It is about self-appreciation and real self-love is built upon a foundation of self-worth. Whereby we feel worthy, where we respect our self and where we are authentically interested, both in our own wellbeing and we are interested in the wellbeing of others.

So loving yourself, in a healthy way, is all about validating oneself as a human being, and part of this real love, which by the way is a selfless love, is that we realize our needs as well as the needs of others.

While many people in society are selfish, many more people are actually burning themselves out by running after everyone else and ignoring their own needs. Fulfilling our own needs and wishes in no way is a selfish thing, so long as we appreciate others and help them in their quest for self-fulfilment too!

Taking a break, having a treat, listening to nice music, going to the beauty parlour or gym, having a hobby or just spending time alone, or with friends are all examples of ways in which we can take time out for ourselves and appreciate and love ourselves. If we don't love ourselves, in a healthy way, then it is not possible to love others. If we feel unworthy and spend our entire time running after everyone else, while ignoring our own needs and wants, then we become frustrated and stressed, which is not good?

In order to appreciate ourselves, and our self-worth, it is a good idea to read some good positive self-help books, listen to inspiring speeches and watch inspiring videos. This is good mind-feed, whereby we boost ourselves and take on a more positive view of the world in which we live.

De-Stress-in

So far, we have looked at some strategies which will help to promote a more relaxed lifestyle and a renewed sense of inner appreciation. But what to do about the very real fact that we are facing stress, every day!

We can't escape it, so what are we going to do about it!

There is a difference between **DISTRESS** on the one hand and **DE-STRESS** on the other. Distress is the common state of modern man, whereas **DE-STRESS** is the answer to our condition of distress!

But how to de-stress?

When it is not possible to avoid stress, when we must face our obligations and get on with things we can still de-stress, do you know how?

Removing Detachment to Stress Results in De-Stress!!!

While we cannot remove our physical bodies from stress, and while we must still be mentally focused, we can at least remove our attachment to the stress. Attachment is the cause of all of our pain. For example, if I stamp my big toe against a chair it will hurt, but if I snub my big toe and then keep on thinking about it, certainly the pain will last longer and be worse. Do you ever notice how when we have small injuries, it is always a better idea to kind of forget about it, that way usually the pain goes away quickly!

Have you ever noticed a headache leaving you?

Probably not, I know I haven't, and I've had lots of headaches over the course of my lifetime. Every time I get a headache, and it goes, it is always a kind of shock to me when it's gone. I have a headache, and its there, then after some time I think about the headache and I suddenly realise that it's gone!

Obviously when our headache goes something has shifted, but not only this, when we forget about our headache our attachment to it dissipates, and so too to some degree the headache itself disappears!

Detachment, from our life's problems, can also be described as having a philosophical attitude. Now some people are born with a very philosophical mind-set, whereby they learn to let go of things and put everything into perspective, but even if you're not born this way you can aspire to be a little bit more philosophical in outlook. Definitely becoming more philosophical is largely an acquired skill.

It is a skill based, upon the development of a certain level of inner awareness, combined with a mental viewpoint that puts things into perspective. Becoming more self-aware and putting things into a better perspective is all easily possible when we spend time regularly reading, listening and watching, material which is good for our minds and our heats.

I know it's not easy, but working towards a more philosophical viewpoint, which is a lifelong activity, is certainly a tactic which will bring about more peace, even in the most stressful conditions, and of course it will realty reduce many negative health effects, one of which been high blood pressure.

Meditation

Meditation is probably the least understood of all activities on this planet. When we think of meditation, an image of some sage like being meditating in a cave or on a rock, in a Buddha pose, comes to mind. And of course people have all these silly ideas about meditation and meditators, such as the mind been free of distractions and meditators somehow being at peace all the time, all of which is nonsense.

First of all, what is meditation?

Meditation is the process of putting one's mind on one point, otherwise known as one pointedness!

That's it!

When we focus on one thing it sharpens our mental capacity and it reduces mental stress. However, meditators are not capable of a thoughtless state (or not for long anyway), and certainly they're just as likely to be as stressed as everyone else.

So why then practice meditation?

Practice meditation because the efforts (note efforts and not necessarily results). The efforts to maintain a one pointed focus produces a grounded state, whereby we become more balanced, we become more at one with ourselves and we become happier. Another interesting side effect, of meditation, is that we become more self-aware. In our present glitzy glamorous world, in which we live, we are getting so defocused because of all the endless external stimulation around us, that we forget to look within. The more we look without, the less happy we are within ourselves and effectively we become, over time, a stranger to ourselves, a sort of puppet on a string, as it were. But who's pulling the string? Everyone and everything, that's the problem that's why we end up with so much distress and heartache!

If we're not pulling our own string, someone else will pull it for us and with disastrous consequences!

So do yourself a favour and getting meditating, you will learn about yourself and who you are and learn to appreciate yourself better, when you sit with yourself, in meditation. After all, when we meditate we are spending time with the most important person in our life, and who is that? Well it's our own self of course! And when we spend time, with ourselves, we get to know and befriend the person who we really are!

But how to meditate?

Meditation is actually easier than you might think. Most people set silly expectations and think that they never meditate because they are always thinking thoughts. Well you will be thinking thoughts as long as live, so don't judge yourself too healthy!

Anytime that we find ourselves focusing on one thing, to the point that we ignore other things, this is a state of meditation. For example, if you are focused on doing some activity and someone calls your name, but you don't hear them, this is meditation. So just get over the picturesque ideas of what meditation is and instead get back to what meditation really is!

One popular meditation technique, which has given meditation a bad rap, is the state of Samadhi. Samadhi is a conscious less state, but it's not sleep! In the 1950's and 1960's, a time when many Indian spiritual teachers came to the west, they tended to emphasize Samadhi, as it is an amazing state. However, Samadhi is just another meditation tool, and a mindless one at that, literally mindless!

Samadhi doesn't really achieve much, but the concept sounds cool. In reality millions of people mediate every day, from many different parts of the world and they struggle with their thoughts, but that's ok. Meditation is not about the end result, rather it's about the activity.

Meditation is not About the End Result Rather it's About the Activity itself!

The activity of trying to focus our mind on one thing, strengthens the mind and this concentration of thought, focuses our consciousness and makes us feel more whole, more complete. The outer attractions, of this world, pull us out of ourselves and we become dilute and vaguely unhappy, while the effort to focus on one thing, brings us back into ourselves and makes us more complete, that's it.

In many ways human consciousness is akin to a beam of light. Pull it back from a surface and it becomes diffuse, scattered; bring it close to a surface and it becomes focused, with laser like precision.

Where is happiness and peace of mind?

There in the focused mind!

Just look at a young child and how happy they are in their little world.

Why is this?

Because they are focused, it's that simple.

So getting back to meditation techniques there are a great many. If you're interested in a spiritual orientated mediation system than take a look at his one heartfullness.com , this is the meditation system which I follow.

If you want a more secular system, than there are a great many books which you can read on the subject and many meditation courses are run all vote the world. I have a couple of articles on my blog which provide a detailed introduction, for anyone who wants to give meditation a try.

The one bit of advice, which I will give, is to avoid any sense of judgement between one system and another. Too many meditators judge their system as greater than another system, which is all rather silly. Just try out some meditation methods, and see what works for you, while respecting other people's beliefs and attitudes towards the subject.

Summing up Lifestyle Changes

We have covered a great range of sub-topics in our overview of lifestyle changes. Everything from diet to exercise, to de-stressing and simplifying our life's and even meditation, as ways of improving our life's and our health. But what has all this got to do with blood pressure?

Well hopefully, by now you are beginning to see that blood pressure is not so much an ailment as rather it's more a case of it been a symptom of an unbalanced life. Now life been complex, as we all know it is, this imbalance is coming from all sorts of avenues. Because of this, when we look at making lifestyle changes, we have to approach it from many different angles!

Men and women are now at odds within themselves and with the world around them. However, returning to some previous ideal age, is both impossible and unwise. Out modern era, while stressful it does express the pinnacle of human achievement. In simple terms we cannot go back, and even if we could we probably would like it much either!

I remember one day when walking with my brother, we walked through a deserted structure built many hundreds of years ago, maybe nearly a thousand years ago, Ireland is full of such structures. Anyhow, we used our imaginations to envisage how these simply stone buildings must have looked all those years ago, and what came to our minds was the sheer physical difficulty of living in that era.

No central heating, no damp protection, no double glazing, hell no windows! It was a wet cold, miserable world, at least on a physical level not to mention witch hunts, internecine wars and plagues!

You can take your ideal ancient life and stick it, I for one am sticking with central heating, air conditioning, TV, internet and smart phones!

So there's no going back, there's only going forward, but going forward is not enough, it's how we go forward that really matters.

We can allow ourselves, to be shot into our respective futures as if out of a canon, misdirected, out of control, clutching for straws. Or we can move forward in a paced manner, moving with the ups and downs of life and adapting as we go, centred and grounded. It is this approach, which will not only help our happiness levels, but also it will improve our health and this of course includes our blood pressure.

Blood pressure is another symptom of imbalance; we need to approach reduction in blood pressure as a lifestyle activity. We have to rebalance our lifestyles and in the process so many things will improve, not just our blood pressure.

Chapter Four - Pranayama

Pranayama is an ancient system of yogic breathing techniques, which hail from India. Pranayama basically consists of various breathing techniques, whereby the inhalation, exhalation and holding of the breath are all modulated, in an effort to stimulate subtle energetic currents within the human body.

In the theory of pranayama, the breath is prana (meaning energy) and this panic energy can be stimulated via breath manipulation. In particular, there are two nerve channels which help move the flow of this panic energy throughout the body. These are Ida and Pingala. Ida is feminine and moves along the left hand side of the body, and this current of energy flows through the left nostril. Pingala, is masculine, it moves along the right hand side of the body and its current circulates via the right nostril. In a balanced physical state, breath will flow smoothly for one hour via the Ida and then for another hour via the Pingala, and this process keeps on repeating throughout the day.

Advanced pranayama's can make amazing changes to this panic energy, and the kundalini energy can be stimulated and made to move up the sushumna channel, which runs along the length of the spinal cord. These advanced pranayama's are extremely dangerous, and should not be attempted without the strict guidance of an advanced pranayama teacher, commonly known as a master or guru of pranayama. These teachers are extremely rare, so be careful if your local yoga teacher tries to teach an advanced pranayama; these advanced techniques can result in terrible nervous and physiological problems. Anyone who is properly, trained in pranayama teaching will more than likely have spent time in India, training directly under a pranayama master, so beware!

For our interest, we are not going to focus on advanced techniques. Rather we will practice several extremely safe pranayama's, which have been proven over time to be safe and highly effective, at reducing blood pressure rates.

Basic Rules and Contraindications

- Always breathe through the nostrils, both for the inhalation and the exhalation also.
- Pranayama should be carried out slowly and sedately and should not be forced. If any discomfort is felt, stop immediately.
- Do not take any stimulant (tea, coffee, alcohol etc., immediately after pranayama practice, as the bodies energies are in a subtle state of balance).
- Pranayama sometimes causes problems for ladies during menstruation. Ladies should experiment, a little, and see if they feel ok doing pranayama during this time, if not then they should skip it for a few days.
- Pregnant ladies should not do agnisara kriya, bahya pranayama or kapalabhati, and they should practice all other pranayama's in a gentle manner.
- High blood pressure patients should practice all pranayama's in a gentle manner.

- In the case of post-surgery patients, they should wait at least one week before attempting pranayama and kapalabhati should be practised only after a period of at least six months after surgery.

A Serious Warning!!!

These are the basic rules and contraindications. Use common-sense and make sure that you feel comfortable, at all times. Pranayama's are the complete opposite of aggressive western styled training. In the west, we are used to intense workouts, and competitive efforts, to beat our own or other people's records. However, in eastern exercise systems it's all about balance and being comfortable.

In particular, pranayama's are the most powerful exercises, which we are covering in this book. Taoist yoga and hatha yoga techniques are all pretty harmless, when compared to pranayama. Breathing is the most powerful activity, in the human body; we can survive weeks without food and days without water, but only minutes without air!

Also in the Indian yogic system of pranayama, they believe in these subtle energy systems, outlined above. Maybe you don't believe in such things, but one thing is for sure, people who mess with pranayama's hurt themselves, while people who are careful often undergo terrific healings.

So be careful and also be aware that this is a very subtle system, and good effects are not dependent upon exertion!

Although pranayama's are potentially hazardous, I am including them in this book because while we are dealing with the most potentially hazardous exercise, they are also the most potentially healing exercises. In particular, pranayama is very effective at reducing or even completely curing high blood pressure. But, it must be cared out gently!

In particular, aggressive exercises like Kapalabhati have received some negative attention, in recent times, because over enthusiastic practitioners were doing relentless repetitions, while pushing their bodies aggressively. Kapalabhati, when practised aggressively shakes up all of the internal organs and can result in cardiovascular damage including damage to the heart itself, when carried out recklessly. Yet the same exercise, if carried out gently has a really good therapeutic effect on BP.

I am writing an extensive warning here, because I am sure that many readers will look up video descriptions of these exercises, on YouTube, and they will try to imitate the aggressive gyrations of the you tubers, whom they see before them. But do please remember, that these people are free from hypertension, so takes my advice here and practice gently. Plus if any discomfort is found stop immediately.

Also frequency is another important factor. For these pranayama's, to be really effective, they should be performed on a daily basis, however, they should not be perfumed for an extended period of time, rather do the specified number of reputations and leave it there. If you like perform the exercises twice a day, if you feel comfortable. If on the other hand, if the stated repetitions feel challenging, then do half or quarter the number of reps. Why matters most is good form and regular practice, do this and good results will come!

Finally pranayama doesn't work for everyone and in some cases it will actually make the blood pressure worse!...

So take a tentative approach, by trying out some basic pranayama's each day and noting down in your journal, the BP prior to and just after the exercise. IF BP levels improve great and if not then maybe consider dropping the pranayama's. Everyone is different and you have to adjust your approach and try to figure out what works for you. The cause of blood pressure is always an energetic deficiency, but while the principles of cause and cure are universal, the actual cure tactics will vary from person to person!

Benefits of Pranayama:

Pranayama has a great many benefits which includes:

- Pranayama reduces hypertension (but some pranayama are contraindicated)
- Pranayama reduces diabetes
- Pranayama reduces asthma
- Pranayama removes free radicals from the body
- Pranayama aids fat loss
- Pranayama improves the metabolism of the body

- Pranayama improves the autonomic nervous system thus aiding digestive functioning, cardiovascular performance and the working of the bowels, glandular system (pineal gland, hypothalamus, pituitary gland, thyroid, thymus, adrenal gland, pancreas and gonads)
- Pranayama reduces stress and aids peace of mind
- Pranayama aids focus and concentration

This list represents a really broad range of positive effects, and from the point of view of reduction in blood pressure rates, pranayama improves not only our blood circulation but it also improves the overall efficiency of our organs and our metabolism. What this means, in simple terms, is that pranayama helps to rebalance our inner physiology, and it is this rebalancing which improves not only our blood pressure rates but also our entire inner health balance, which is a really good thing.

Medical Research Confirms the Effectiveness of Pranayama's

Quite a bit of research has been carried out on the effectiveness of pranayama's, and many of them have been demonstrated to reduce high blood pressure.

Sukha Pranayama: In a scientific research program (http://www.ncbi.nlm.nih.gov/pubmed/22398346), they took twenty three hypertensive patients and made them practise this deep breathing technique, for five minute periods. At the end of each five minute practice period, their blood pressure reduced significantly (approximately by 5%). A five percent reduction in blood pressure rates is really good. While more research has to be carried out, in order to assess the long-term effects of sukha pranayama, initial results suggest a good potential reduction, if practised regularly.

Bhastrika Pranayama (Slow Paced): In this research, using bhastrika pranayama, at a slow pace(for hypertensives this technique must be performed slowly and gently, otherwise it will worsen the blood high pressure condition), they found that after each session, both the systolic and diastolic rates reduced by approximately 5% (115.43+/-10.79 systolic moving down to 107.84+/-9.85 and diastolic reducing down from 77.23+/-7.50 down to 73.17 +/- 6.53), plus their average heart rate reduced noticeably, which in turn should have a good effect on blood pressure rates. This study can be seen here: http://www.ncbi.nlm.nih.gov/pubmed/19249921

Pranava Pranayama: In this study (http://www.ncbi.nlm.nih.gov/pubmed/23734443), 29 obese patients, who had all undergone, at least three years of, hypertensive treatment where divided into a "sham group", who practiced a made up relaxed breathing exercise and a practice group, who practised pranava pranayama. At the end of the study, the "sham group" saw a slight improvement in systolic, diastolic and heart rate, whilst the practice group saw a big reduction in their systolic rates from 134.3 ± 3.8 down to 124.7 ± 3.2; diastolic went down from 77.2 ± 1.3 to 74.9 ± 1.2, and heart rate also dropped down from 77.5 ± 3.3 to 75.3 ± 3.1. Importantly, in this study, the "sham group" had a slight improvement, such as a drop in diastolic from 77.4 ± 2.2 to 76.9 ± 1.6, but this is statistically insignificant, been less than a 1% reduction in diastolic rate, versus the practice group who saw a 3% reduction. So even taking into account a possibility of placebo effect, whereby the positive thinking of the patient brings around some degree of success, the success rate is still very small (less than 1%).

Furthermore, what would be the combined effect of a hypertensive patient pursuing all three methods outlined above?

It is a synergistic effect, whereby over a period of weeks, the cumulative effect of each breathing technique, slowly rebalances various processes within the body.

High blood pressure, basically occurs when the body starts to get out of balance. This process occurs over time, but usually the patient will only know about it when some problem occurs, which means that the actually aetiology (cause), had probably started years earlier. So by the time we have developed symptoms, a series of imbalances has already taken place. With pranayama, each of these techniques quickly rebalances, some of these processes,

Another thing, which we can take from this research, is that even a few minutes of pranayama will produce a statistically significant result, where the hypertensive patient will feel immediate relief. This is a great thing, as for example, an obese person has to wait weeks before they see a noticeable reduction in fat, but with pranayama's, noticeable positive results are available within minutes. This is particularly useful, if say you are having a stressful day and your blood pressure is unusually high. Five to fifteen minutes will produce a noticeable reduction in the effects of this high BP, and that's a really useful thing to know!

How to perform the Pranayama's

Seating

Cobra Pose

(courtesy of Jesús Bonilla (Tanumânasî)

Cross Legged Pose

(Courtesy of wiki How)

Sitting in a Chair Pose

(Picture courtesy of wiki How)

Sukha Pranayama

Sukha pranayama is probably the easiest of all yogic breathing exercises, to perform.

1. Sit comfortable, with back straight. You can sit either cross legged, on folded legs or even in a chair, so long as your back is straight. A straight back is necessary, in order to feel the beneficial effects of yogic breathing. One of the problems, of the modern era, is that we tend to slump, and this results in shallow breathing, which in turn causes our blood to be deoxygenated. Naturally, if our blood is deoxygenated, we will lack some energy, and over time ill health will kick in. Sitting

straight and breathing fully, is probably one of the easiest and most beneficial life's changes, which we can make, in order to rebalance our health!

2. Start breathing slowly, inhaling to a count of four. Slowly, like this...1...2...3...4
3. Then immediately start exhaling, to the exact same rhythm of 1...2...3...4
4. Repeat twelve times (or whatever feels comfortable, stress should be avoided)

Benefits of Sukha Pranayama

- Lowers blood pressure
- Relaxes both body and mind
- Improves concentration
- Reliefs psychological stress and emotional depression

Bhastrika Pranayama (Slow Paced)

Bhastirka is by far one of the most powerful pranayama's which you can perform. However, IT IS POTENTIALLY HAZARDOUS, and this is the case for two reasons. First of all, if performed in the normal manner, it requires a rigorous shaking of the body which can in turn damage the internal organs. Secondly, if practised for too long, a period, it can once again cause internal damage. The key with all yoga pranayama's is to perform them in such a manner that there is no stress. This is the opposite of western styled physical training, where people are going for the burn etc. With yoga pranayama's however we are looking for a subtle movement of energy through the body, which gently rebalances everything, consequently aggressive approaches are to be avoided, and in particular so in this exercise. Rather perform it slowly and carefully.

Bhastrika means "bellows breathe", so the image which comes to mind is of the lungs operating like a giant blacksmiths bellows, inflating a little slowly and then expelling with great force and speed. As hypertensive patients however, we are going to inhale longer and exhale for a shorter period, but without the aggressive pumping action of traditional bhastrika.

1. Sit in an erect posture. Traditionally it should be a crossed legged position, however, even a sitting position is fine as long as your back remains erect.
2. Inhale through the nose (always inhale and exhale through the nose).
3. Breathe in deeply and breathe out very quickly. The in breath must be longer then the outbreath.
4. Breathing should be quick (because bhastrika pranayama can be contraindicated in hypertensive cases breathe quickly but not aggressively, for people who are free of high blood pressure the breathing process can be more aggressive, meaning jerking the body during the inhalation process).
5. Perform ten breaths (inhalation and exhalation) quickly.
6. Take a break of a few seconds then begin another round of 10 breaths.
7. Repeat four rounds, as long as it feels comfortable to do so.

The principle behind bhastrika is to force more oxygen into the body, via the longer inhalations and to expel impurities via very short bursting exhalations.

There are many benefits to bahstrika pranayama, which includes:

- Reduction in blood pressure
- Increased oxygenation of the blood, which replenishes every cell in the body
- Increased energy levels
- Improved digestion
- Elevation of asthmatic conditions
- Purification of the nerves, which improves panic energy flow throughout the body
- Spiritual upliftment

To fully understand the benefits of bhastrika, it is necessary to practice for a little while. But do remember that it is a very powerful exercise. In order to prevent any damage, to the cardiovascular system and lungs, it is vitally important that the following precautions be followed:

i) Do not force
ii) Start gently and speed up gradually in a manner whereby exertion is not felt
iii) Do not practice beyond four rounds per sitting, and do no more than two sittings per day

If you Google bhastrika pranayama, a lot of videos will appear, especially in YouTube, of various yogis's performing aggressive and fast variations of this exercise. But do remember that these are experienced exponents of yoga. As a beginner, and particular as a hypertensive patient, restraint is required. We are looking for a gently stimulation of the lungs in this exercise, no force, just enough to get some vitality going. Start carefully and increase gently over time!

Panava Pranayama

Panava comes from the Sanskrit word 'OM' and in this exercise variations on the 'om' sound are made, in order to enhance the health of the body. In yogic science a great deal of study has been carried out on the effects of sound and the psychic system. In this pranayama, we will be using two breathing techniques and humming two yogic sounds in order to stimulate the healing process.

1. Sit in an erect position
2. Close your eyes
3. Put the hands into the 'Gyan mudra' position (whereby the forefinger and thumb meet).
4. Place your hands in the 'Gyan mudra 'position on your thighs.
5. Breathe in deeply, while focusing upon the lower section of your lungs.
6. Breath out, making the sound 'aaaahhhhhhh'.
7. This energises the lower body, legs, hips and pelvic organs.

8. Then in the second part of this exercise we are going to make the chinmaya mudra. In this case we join the forefinger to the thumb, while closing the other fingers, as if forming a fist.
9. Once again place the hand, now this time in 'Chinmaya mudra' position onto your thighs.
10. Breathe in deeply, while focusing upon the mid chest region...
11. Exhale, but this time say 'ooooooohhhhhhhhhh' during the outbreath
12. This mudra concentrates the panic energy into the mid chest region, thus repansihes on the heart region.

GYAN MUDRA

CHINMAYA MUDRA

Benefits of panama Pranayama

There are many benefits of this pranayama, which includes the following:

- Reduction of high blood pressure levels
- Improvement of heart related problems
- Improvement in blood and energy flow to the lower body
- Improvement in heart health
- Reduces anger and anxiety

- Cures insomnia
- Cures migraines
- Helps reduce paralysis

Chapter Five - Hatha Yoga

Savasanna

Savasanna, otherwise known as the corpse pose, is without doubt the easiest hatha yoga pose, which can be performed. In Savasanna, the practitioner simply lies on their back with their legs and arms stretched outward, as if in a five star formation. While, it is very simple, do not underestimate it's effectiveness, as it is designed to greatly reduce physical stress and its effect on blood pressure levels is easily noted, as blood pressure always ties into physical stress levels.

1. Lie on your back with arms and legs outstretch at a 45 degree angle.
2. Maintain hands in an open upturned pose.
3. Relax and breathe deeply.
4. Stay in this position for five to ten minutes

Paschimottanasana (Forward Bend Pose)

Paschimottanasana, is a very simple yet effective asana (posture). It can be difficult to perform it to its full extent, but do not worry if you find yourself only able to complete half the stretch, as over time flexibility will increase. The important thing is to give the legs and back a good stretch. In the process of doing so blood flow to the middle of the body will increase and in particular the lower back and hamstrings.

Regardless how deep you get into the posture, do hold the final position for a few seconds in order to allow the increased blood flow to do its work.

Benefits:

- Relieves blood pressure
- Sooths anxiety
- Promotes calmness

- Relaxes nerves
- Reduces fatigue
- Reduces sinusitis
- Good for ovaries and uterus
- Good for kidneys and liver
- Good for spinal health
- Relieves insomnia
- Improves digestion

Technique

1. Sit on the floor with legs outstretched.
2. Ease arms directly above the head.
3. Stretch the hands and arms downwards towards the toes. If possible clasp the soles of the feet and hold this stretch for five seconds. If this is not possible then simply stretch to whatever is comfortable for you.
4. Release and once again sit upright
5. Repeat eight times.

Contraindications:

- Do not practice in case of a herniated disc.
- It might not be appropriate for some pregnant ladies.
- Avoid if suffering from hip problems
- Avoid if suffering from sciatica.

Photo Courtesy of Joseph RENGER
(https://commons.wikimedia.org/wiki/File:Paschimottanasana.jpg#filelinks)

Shashankasana (hare pose) and Balasana Pose (Pose of a Child)

Both of these are simple poses whereby the practitioner sits on their knees. In the case of balasana, the body is folded and the arms rest at ones side, whereas with shashankasana, the arms are outstretched in front.

Benefits:

Both poses have similar benefits to Paschimottanasana, in that they involve the bending forward of the body, which stimulates the spine and inner organs. Also, all of these postures are extremely relaxing, and this is the main thing, from the point of view of reducing blood pressure levels. The benefits come from increased blood flow and energetic flow via the reflow of panic energy.

Shashankasana provides a better stretch than balasana, so really it's a case of trying both and seeing which one works best for you.

Techniques

1. Sit on your knees.
2. In balasana, rest the weight of your upper body upon your legs, whereby the chest rests on the thighs and let the head rest on the floor, while the arms are on the sides.
3. In the case so shashankasana, begin the same but instead of placing arms on your side, stretch them out in front instead.
4. Hold the position for a comfortable time period. Stat with thirty seconds and work up to two minutes. Don't worry about repetitions, rather make yourself comfortable and stay there while comfortable, then sit back up again then resume after a few seconds. In total two or three repetitions, with extended time periods where the pose is held, is ideal.

SHASHANKASANA

Photo Courtesy of https://vikasacharya.wordpress.com/2015/06/13/how-the-yoga-asana-helps-in-fertility/

An Important Note on Performing Yoga Asanas

Yoga asanas are incredibly helpful, at rebalancing the body, and as a consequence of this they are an effective way to heal oneself. However, for anyone who has not tried hatha yoga before, it can come as a real shock when exercises, which appear easy to perform, turn out to be especially challenging. The thing to remember, with hatha yoga postures, is that there is a presumption that the practitioner is already in good health!

It must be remembered, that for many thousands of years most people where physically active and hence had fairly good flexibility levels. The original creators of hatha yoga, developed these postures, at a time, when the general populace where busy working in physical jobs and so already had well-toned, flexible physiques. Also, back in ancient India most people did not use chairs, indeed chairs are a recent feature of Indian life, and many younger Indians still like to sit on the floor rather than the chair. Chairs, while been a great invention, limit the range of hip motion and consequently people who sit on chairs a lot, have restricted hip mobility.

All of these factors add up to make even the most basic yoga asanas, difficult for many people to perform today. The exercises, listed above, have been picked because of their relative ease, but still some degree of difficulty might initially be felt, particularly in physically heavier people and older people.

Do not worry, if for now, you cannot complete these poses. The traditional approach, to mastering yoga asanas, is to begin slowly and do the best you can without straining. Practice daily and observe over time an increase in flexibility. The key is to practice daily and even the more difficult poses can be mastered. Stick with it for a few weeks, and the poses mentioned above will become far more doable, within a few weeks.

Also, perform the asanas slowly and deliberately. Trying to concentrate, on the movement and focus on good form, these are not western calisthenics, which need to be rushed through in order to get the burn. Rather they need to be applied slowly and with complete awareness, this will give the internal organs the necessary gentle message, which is necessary in order to see good, progressive and safe results!

Traditional Chinese Poises

Traditional Chinese Medicine dates back to around 3500 years, but along the way it became inextricably linked with Taoism. Taoism (pronounced as Daoism) was initially founded by the famous Chinese philosopher, Lao Tzu. Lau Tzu wrote the famous book 'Tao Te Ching', which basically means 'The way', the Tao(dao) meaning way. Interestingly Lau Tzu's work and subsequent Taoist works have focused upon the philosophical aspects of traditional Chinese thought, and over time these philosophical concepts would make their way back into the ancient traditional Chinese medical treatments.

These ancient Chinese therapeutics , have over time diversified into such training systems as Tai Chi, Chi Ghong, Wu shu and also as Taoist health techniques, which are sometimes known as Taoist yoga (which is actually a misnomer, as yoga is distinctly Indian in character).

Some of these systems focus on very difficult, and sometimes rather esoteric practices, but by and far the majority of them are focused on very easy exercises, which gently balance the health of the practitioner.

I am adding some of the more gentle variations of these exercises, as they work really well and are easy to perform.

The Crane, The Turtle and the Solar Plexus Exercises

If you Google these exerises, a few options will come up and most of them are difficult to perform. However, exercises of the same name but which are easy to perform, and at the same time are very beneficial, have already been popularised back in the early 1980's by Stephen T Chang and his famous books on Taoist healing techniques. I like these particular variations because of their simplicity and effectiveness. There are lots of interesting exercises, out there, but which are difficult to perform, and really it's not necessary to wrap your legs around your head, in order to heal your body. Rather, many exercises which originate from taoist healing systems, are very easy to perform and should be popularised once again because they really are that good.

Crane

Starting with the Crane, it is named in deference to the crane bird which sucks its abdomen in towards its back bone when standing. A simple variation of this is to simply lie on your back and breath. Breath out while trying to suck your navel back in towards your spine, then breath in and literarily fill up your abdomen until it bloats outward, almost as if it's about to burst. Sucking ones abdomen inwards massages the stomach and intestines, while breathing very deeply into the abdomen charges the stomach with air. Young babies practice abdominal breathing, whilst most adults perform superficial breathing via the top of their lungs, breathing from the abdomen is the natural way to breath. Filling the abdomen first and then the lungs results in a really deep and beneficial breath.

Benefits

The crane has several benefits, which includes the following:

- Strengthening the stomach (which aids digestion and energy production)
- Massaging the intestines (which aids digestion and energy production and prevents constipation)
- Deep breathing stimulates the nervous system and oxygenates the blood (which in turn reduces blood pressure)
- Deep breathing combined with deep exhalations extract toxins from the blood
- Deep inhalations combined with deep exhalations, carried out with conscious intent promotes yang energy (active energy) in the body.

Technique

1. Lie down.
2. Breath out, while sucking in your abdomen, focus upon the navel retracting towards the spinal cord. Go as far as is comfortable and then squeeze slightly. This process can then be enhanced by pressing gently downwards, with the palms of your hands.
3. When fully exhaled immediately inhale, by breathing into the abdomen and filling up your belly until it fills like its ready to explode. At this stage the breath will naturally fill the lungs from the lower position. Hold for a few seconds and then exhale once again.
4. Repeat this process of exhalation followed by deep inhalation and continue for about five minutes in total.

It is important, with this exercise to carry it out gently. Do not force, rather gently exhale and gently inhale. Also, there is a good chance that some slight discomfort will be felt during the exhalation. This is fine, the reason for this, is because most of us have backed up faeces, within our intestines. Which is a common, side effect of highly processed foods, and lack of fibre in our diet. Keep with the program and gently massage the lower intestines, by gently squeezing (but not forcing) the lower intestines.

With this exercise, blood will gently seep into the microvilli of the lower intestines, which in turn will aid digestion and health in general.

What has this exercise got to do with high blood pressure?

This is a great exercise for building up the two most important organs of the body, from the point of view of health and vitality. A strong stomach will break down food efficiently, while strong clean intestines will effectively absorb nutrients into the body. The effect of these two organs been boosted is an improved immune system, higher vitality levels and improved yang (active) energy, which in turn helps to balance blood pressure naturally.

The Solar Plexus Exercise

Like Stephen T Chang, I am a great believer in this exercise, although the way I do it differs considerable from his method. The way I recommend doing this exercise is twofold, it involes massaging the solar plexus and also using visualisation exercises.

From a nervous point of view, the solar plexus is a major nerve group, within the body. The solar plexus is found at the base of the sternum. Lie down and poke this area with your finger, when a sudden stabbing pain is felt, then bingo!..this is the solar plexus. From a TCM point of view, the solar plexus represents the emotional brain, while the physical brain is simply a computing machine. Whenever we feel upset or overwhelmed, we feel discomfort in the solar plexus. Stage nerves, when we have to step up and speak in front of others and feeling nauseous when facing an interview, are obvious examples of an overwhelmed solar plexus. Also, in the case of kids, often their stomach aches are actually caused by emotional overwhelming feelings, in the solar plexus and massaging will often help greatly.

The solar plexus is really important, because our bodies are designed for a far more simple era, consequently, we often feel overwhelmed because we are designed for simple living.

Solar plexus exercises, will greatly help to calm down anxious feelings and obviously this will help blood pressure levels because of the feelings of rejuvenation which come from this exercise, since often high blood pressure levels are created by tension and feelings of being overwhelmed. So this is a great deep relaxation exercise.

Technique

1. Lie down.
2. Locate the solar plexus and begin massaging it in a clockwise manner. This is particularly useful when feeling hurt feelings and anxious feelings. If general fatigue is felt, but emotions are not disturbed then just jump ahead to the next stage.
3. Hold both hands either side of the solar plexus and then visualise divine white light (or egg yolk yellow, if you like – as this is the astral colour of the solar plexus chakra) gently filling the solar plexus.
4. Maintain this position and occasionally remind oneself of the light. Continue for five to fifteen minutes.

Also, if you like soft music can be played along while this gently recharging process is taking place.

Turtle

The turtle is a simple exercise, yet it is a great way to relax the neck and shoulders, which in turn brings about relaxation and consequently this de-stressing effect promotes relief of high blood pressure.

Benefits

1. Stretches the spine.
2. Relaxes the shoulders and neck.
3. Boosts the thyroid and parathyroid.
4. Boosts the metabolism.
5. Boosts inner energy delivery within the body.

Tecnhique

1. Sit (cross legged or on a chair).
2. Bring your chin down to your chest and slowly inhale. The neck will feel slightly stretched while the shoulders will relax deeply.
3. Slowly lift the head upwards and backwards, until the back of the head touched the atlas joint, at the back of the neck. Exhale while doing so, this time the throat will feel stretched.
4. Repeat twelve times, but do not strain.

Contraindications

In general this is a very safe exercise but do bear in mind that for someone who suffers from serious neck injuries or scoliosis, for example, might feel pain and it might be damaging. So obviously, use your common sense. No discomfit should be felt either during or after this exercise. If any discomfort if felt, do stop immediately!

Various Massages and Rubbings for Lower Blood Pressure

There are several great massages, and rubbings, which instantly reduce blood pressure levels and which are easy and quick to perform.

1. Kidney energy is really important, from the point of view of overall health and wellbeing, in the body, and it just so happens that we have a really good kidney acupressure point on the soles of our feet. This point kidney 1, when pressed, first thing in the morning will easily boost energy levels and energetic balance within the body.
2. The trick is to knead this point (as in squeeze and rub deeply, at one and the same time).
3. Continue for 100 times (about 2 minutes).

Head and Neck massage

1. Start massaging from the forehead till the vertex (top of the head) and occipital region (back of the head).
2. Then turn the palms inwards and massage with the lateral aspect of the fingers the bilateral hypotensive grooves behind the ears and gallbladder 20 (which is located at the base of the skull- in the depression between the sternocleidomastoid and the trapezius muscles).
3. Finally, massage along the sides of the neck and down to the upper chest while gently pushing and caressing the carotid artery with the lateral aspect of the back of the hands.
4. Repeat twenty times in total.

Chapter Six - Herbal Cures

Walnuts and Honey

Walnuts and honey are one of the best remedies for high blood pressure and cardiovascular health. Also, unlike most natural remedies, walnuts and honey tastes delicious! It's like either a base or a topping for cheesecake and while eating it a pang of guilt comes that surely this must be bad rather than good for health?

But nothing could be further from the truth.

Benefits of Walnuts

1. Lowers cholesterol
2. Reduces inflammation
3. Prevents erratic heart arrhythmias
4. Reduces plaque formation in the arteries
5. Reduces cardiovascular risk
6. Prevents cancer and bacterial growths
7. Boosts the immune system
8. Improves cognitive function
9. Maintains bone health
10. Prevents gallstones
11. Kills intestinal parasites

12. Aids weight loss

This is quite a list. In particular walnuts are a good source of the essential amino acid L-arginine, which improves the elasticity of arteries. Also, walnuts possess omega 3 acid which in turn which reduces cholesterol and arteriosclerosis and heart attack risk.

Benefits of Honey

1. Reduces blood pressure
2. Good for energy
3. Good for blood
4. Anti-bacterial
5. Aids digestion
6. High in antioxidants
7. Anti-cancerous properties
8. Boosts the immune system

Try this formula out on a daily basis. It tastes great and will aid cardiovascular health while reducing blood pressure naturally!

Cinnamon

Cinnamon possesses many great health effects which include:

- High in anti-inflammatory properties

- High in antioxidants

- Good for heart health

- Great for diabetics

- Helps brain health

- Fights bacterial infections

- Anti-cancer compound

- Good for fighting digestive fungi (ex candida)

- Fights allergies

Although cinnamon is an amazing product for reducing blood sugar levels in diabetics, it also works well as a hypertensive, In a study of 58 diabetic patients, as well as reducing blood sugar levels, they noted a drop in average diastolic blood pressure levels from an median of 85.2 down to 80.2, which is around a 6% drop on blood pressure levels, simply by taking a few grams of cinnamon every day!10 And another great benefit of cinnamon, was a noted improvement in triglyceride levels (which are the unhealthy fats which encourage the build-up of plaque in the arteries), which means that cinnamon helps to reduce cholesterol levels naturally!

How to take Cinnamon

A minimum of 2 grams a day produces a good effect.

Cinnamon in Food: Cinnamon can be added to our cooking or in our herbal teas or even in our baking efforts.

Cinnamon Capsules: Cinnamon can be taken in capsule form.

Cinnamon Tea

1. Add two or three cinnamon sticks to 250ml of water
2. Boil and leave to simmer for 10 minutes
3. Strain and serve, adding in lemon and honey for taste.

Garlic

Garlic is a great all round tonic for health and vitality and amongst its many benefits it can boast the following:

- Garlic helps to cure both colds and flu's
- Garlic reduces blood glucose levels
- Garlic protects against dementia of the brain

- Garlic detoxifies the body
- Garlic makes the bones stronger
- Garlic fights allergies
- Garlic is an anti-cancer agent
- Garlic reduces blood pressure levels
- Garlic reduces cholesterol levels
- Garlic protects heart health

In a meta-analysis study, which covered research of the effect of garlic on blood pressure levels, in various studies, over a 50 year period noted an average result of a drop of 7.3+/-1.5mg in the diastolic reading!11

How to Take Garlic

Garlic is one of the most popular herbs in the world and is used very widely as a culinary herb. So chances are that you are already using garlic. However, to get a good benefit from garlic you need to take a good amount of garlic each day. In a study, which observed the effect of various dosages of garlic, noted a result which kept on trending upwards with the greater quantity of garlic taken per day. They measured from 300mg a day up to 1.5mg a day and noted a reduction in blood pressure levels of around 9.5% on average.12

So you can take garlic in your food, as in cooked, or raw or in capsule form but as for quantity I would suggest at least 3 or 4 cloves a day, which is anywhere from 9 to 12 grams of garlic a day. This sounds like a lot, but the active ingredient in garlic is an organo-suplur compound called allicin and the amount varies from garlic clove to garlic clove. So to make sure you are getting a good effect, take several clove of garlic a day!

Ginger

Ginger is another great tonic, which cure many health conditions including:

- Strengthens the immune system
- Cure nausea
- Improves osteoarthritic symptoms
- Improves blood sugar levels in diabetics
- Improves digestion
- Protects against dementia
- Reduces pre-menstrual tension symptoms
- Boosts energy levels
- Reduces high blood pressure

- Reduces cholesterol levels

Ginger helps to reduce cholesterol levels (13), which in turn will protect heart health and in research on the activity of ginger, they noted that it worked in the same way as a calcium channel blocking blood pressure medication, such as amlodiprine, nicardipine and verapamail, for example. 14

So from a clinical scientific point of view, it has been proven that ginger helps to reduce blood pressure levels. On a practical level we can actually witness the yang energy (active energy) improvement which takes place while taking ginger. Ginger is an amazing tonic and when we take it, it heats up our body, recharging us and balancing various subtle energies within our bodies.

From a TCM point of view, high blood pressure always leads back to low yang Qi energy levels, so ginger been a great yang Qi tonic, means that ginger is one of the most vital blood pressure lowering herbs which you can take.

However, in some cases, it is contraindicated!

Contraindications:

The opposite side of yang energy is yang energy, which is the nurturing energy. While high blood pressure levels are created by yang Qi deficiency, in some case if an individual's yang energy levels are very low, then a yang tonic might actually make for an even greater disharmony.

Atypical symptoms of yang deficiency is a dark red collared tongue, with little or no coating on it, a feeling of heat even when the weather is cool, a tendency towards sweating, an inability to sleep, an anxious mood, and often a low level paranoia. If you feel some or all of these symptoms, then observe yourself while taking ginger. If it makes you feel good they fine, but if it makes you feel hotter and more anxious, then stop taking it as in some rare cases it can create an imbalance.

How to Take Ginger

Just like garlic ginger is a very common herb. The easiest way to take ginger is as a tea.

Ginger Tea

1. Take about 5 grams of raw garlic (peel of the outer skin) and then add to about 250ml of water.

2. Boil and leave to simmer for 10 minutes.

3. Then strain and serve while mixing with lemon and honey for taste.

4. You can re-use the ginger later the same day by taking the remnants of garlic and mixing them in an electrical mix with 250ml of water (per cup). Then once again boil, simmer and serve.

Ginger is slow to release its essence, so it has to be boiled for a long time, although when mixed in an electrical blender it releases a lot of its healing compounds. I find by doing this, that the second time I take it that it's stronger than the first. But I leave the electrical mixing until the second time, so as to get more mileage out of the ginger!

To be effective the ginger should be so strong as to burn the back of the throat a little bit. It might not be as tasty as it is very strong, but boy is it powerful!

Maintenance is 1 mug a day and for making an impact with blood pressure opt for 2 to 3 mugs a day!

Cardamom

Cardamom is another common herb and it benefits include:

- Fights mouth bacteria
- Improves breath smell
- Kills toothache!
- Helps digestion
- Detoxiciant
- High in antioxidants

- Anti-pathogenic
- Fights cold and flu
- Fights depression
- Anti-inflammatory
- Diuretic
- Hiccup cure
- Prevents blood clots
- Lowers blood pressure levels

Cardamom has many great benefits which includes lowering blood pressure. In a study on its blood pressure lowering effects they noted a reduction from a diastolic level of 112.59+/-1.77 down to 97.99+/-2.00, so approximately a reduction of 8.7% in blood pressure elvels.15

How to Take Cardamom

One way to take cardamom is to simple chew the cardamom seeds. The outer husk is hard and will have to be spit out, but inside are very small seeds which can be chewed and swallowed. Cardamom is the ultimate toothache cure, so forget about chewing cloves; also it cleanses the mouth and freshens the breath, so simply crewing is a good way to go, other than that cardamom, can be made into a tea.

Cardamom/ Ginger/Cinnamon/Lemon/Honey Tea

1. Cardamom can be boiled on its own and made into a tea but it's a little bit boring. A great option for anyone with high blood pressure is top mix in around 5 grams of ginger (per mug) with two pieces of cinnamon and 2 cardamom seeds with 250 ml of water (per mug). Then boil and leave to simmer for 10 minutes.

2. Strain and serve, adding lemon and phoney for extra health and taste!

Looking at ginger, garlic, cinnamon and cardamom, each one has a significant effect on blood pressure elves, so by imbibing this beverage two to three times a day, will make a significant synergistic effect upon lowering blood pressure levels!

Rauvolfia Serpentina

Rauvolfia Serpentina (snakeroot) is a really powerful root which comes from Asia. Snakeroot is a famous cure for snake bite and is a popular yang Qi tonic in China; also it has a good effect on lowering blood pressure levels.

Snakeroot can be either taken as a powered mixed with water or if you can get your hands on raw snakeroot (as a root, simply take a few small pieces of root, or one big piece and leave overnight in 100ml (3 ounces) of water. Strain and serve and then refill with water and then take again at night time. So ideally it should be taken twice a day.

By far serpent root is the most powerful herb mentioned in this chapter. It will very likely reduce blood pressure levels by at least a good 10 percent, and of course if used along with the other herbs mentioned within, will result in a very noticeable reduction in blood pressure levels.

While this is all good, serpent root is so strong that I feel it is a good idea to cycle on and off serpent root. Rauviolfia serpentina is an excellent herb to take for anyone who has blood pressure which is reluctant to go down and whereby long-term medication appears to be a necessity. The problem with taken allopathic medications, for a long time, is that over a period of months and in some times years, side effects develop and also the medication slowly becomes ineffective resulting in the patient having to change blood pressure medications, anywhere from every six months to every couple of years.

Since Rauvolfia Serpentina is so powerful, that it can often replace the allopathic drugs so that you can come of off the allopathic medication, for a few months, and then after a while cycle back of off the serpent root and back onto the allopathic medicine. The benefit here is that it prevent long –term side effects from developing, with the allopathic drug, and at the same can also be said for serpent root, which being an extreme yang herb, may have an overheating effect upon the body, over a long period of time!

So cycling is a great way to keep both herb and drug from developing side effects or from becoming ineffective.

Finally in the case of a person who has sever hypertension, getting back to an ok level of blood pressure, may end up been very difficult even with the help of drugs. In this case serpent root can go a long way towards normalising blood pressure levels, when combined with allopathic drugs over a long period of time!

Conclusion – Putting it All Together

Ok so we've covered a lot of ground and right about now you might be wondering how to initiate a successful plan.

The idea behind the material, which has been presented in this book, has not been to create a cookie cutter plan but rather to provide you the reader with two things, which are:

A). A theoretical overview which will help you to see how high blood pressure could have developed in the first place.

B). Various resources which you can use at your leisure, experimenting where you go, dropping what does not work and keeping up with that which does work!

So my advice to you is to start by investing in a blood pressure kit and take daily readings, so as to see how you are doing.

Secondly, if you have time read through the chapters on theory and also on lifestyle, and see where you are perhaps burning the candles at both ends. There's no point in doing exercises or in taking herbs while your lifestyle is out of whack. Rather perform a quick itinerary of your life, and see how you can go about balancing different aspects of life better. Getting the basics right, is the first step towards improving blood pressure levels.

The next stage is to pick out an exercise or two, which appears doable in your eyes. It might be a hatha yoga asana or a Taoist yoga asana, for example, it really doesn't matter. Just try out a few of these exercises and see what feels relatively easy. After you complete the require reps check in briefly with your body and see how you feel. This might appear strange, as so many of us are so disconnected from our bodies that we have no idea as to what is good or bad for our health!

Our bodies intrinsically know what's good for them and are quick to give us subtle hints, as to how such a lifestyle choice works either positively or negatively. However, from early childhood we are groomed to like certain foods and lifestyle choices, and over a period of time we forget to listen to our bodies. An example of this disconnect is easily demonstrably with food. We might love a certain type of food, but 20 minutes after we eat it we feel bad. The reason why we like this food, in the first place, is because of deconditioning and then we are driven by our taste buds to go have some more of this food. However, after the food ends up in the stomach, the body now has to deal with it and if the food is toxic or difficult to absorb, then our body responds accordingly. Thus we often enjoy certain things but feel ill after wards, thus indicating a dislike from our body and an liking from our conditioning!

So our bodies communicate in a subtle way and our body never lies! Our body has no ego; rather it simply lets us know what is good or bad for our health. So when you do your exercise, just focus for a few seconds afterwards and try and feel... how do you feel better or worse?

Ideally keep a journal and write in the date and note what exercise you performed and how it made you feel. With a little bit of trial and error and some observation from your side, you should within a few days, have at least one or two exercises which work really well for you. For now continue with these exercises and also add in some herbs.

What herbs to add in?

All of the herbs mentioned above are good, but start of by taking one or two and make a point of taking the correct dosage every day. It takes three weeks to from a habit, so for now maintain maybe two exercises and two herbs and keep going with them for 21 days. After 21 days has passed add in another herb and possibly another exercise or yoga pranayama.

The approach, which I am suggesting here is an easy going, explorative approach, whereby we make slow changes and keep on updating our approach, over a period of weeks and months. There are two good reasons for this, which are:

i. It takes time to learn a new habit or exercise, or in the case of herbs, it takes a few weeks to see the effects, so it makes sense to give each new change a chance to work properly.

ii. It takes 21 days to make a new habit, so it makes sense to keep practicing this new activity so that it becomes natural and normal for us to perform it.

I know that this approach might appear slow, but it's slow and steady which wins the race. The internet is full of blood pressure correcting protocols, but this is all silly. As noted in earlier chapters, your increased blood pressure, has taken time to develop and always a fairly complex aetiology will be found behind the condition, hence a quick cookie cutter protocol might provide some relief but it will only be a shadow of what could be achieved, by creating a comprehensive and holistic program based upon making your own concerted effort to see what works for you.

And this is something which we must realise. While we may have the same symptoms as someone else, more often than not the exact cause and hence exact cure will vary from person to person, so some experimentation is required.

Furthermore, there are lots of great health books out there, but how much of this good advice is actively followed? Not a lot I can assure you!

I remember back in 2009, when I started getting into the idea of rejuvenating myself via exercises, herbs and lifestyle changes. I took out a hard back note book and created an extensive list of what to do. When I started my program, I found that it was taken me one and a half hours a day to complete the program and also that the program was not proofing to be very effective. After a couple of months, I ended up giving up on the program and over the next few years I ended up revisiting this plan several times and in several different ways.

How did I go wrong?

I went wrong by biting off more than I could chew. Everything in a book or on the internet appears easy and exciting. But in reality it often takes a good few attempts at an exercise or making a recipe before we get it right. Secondly, benefits of said exercise will vary from individual to individual and also upon how good you are at performing the exercises. So just running through the motions makes for zero effect on health. Spending an hour and a half a day, going through the motions is simply a waste of our time!

I have learned from my mistakes and now suggest to you to take a more mature approach. Take up a certain exercise or two and add in a herb or two and spend a few weeks getting used to perfmoning them and milking them work for you. When you feel comfortable then add in more.

I suggest that you begin with exercises and herbs, but add in pranayama's a little more slowly as they can be difficult to learn and also pranayama's don't work great for everybody. Basically the hatha yoga and Taoist yoga asana, will definitely help your blood pressure levels, but pranayama's might work for one-person but not another. I have added in the chapter on pranayama, so as to provide you with a resource, but there is a lot of variation in response. If pranayama doesn't work for you then drop it. So starting out asana work well and herbs work really well.

Finally another thing to realise is that we have gotten used to taking pharmaceutical pills send expect instant results. Well herbs take a week or two to work and so do most asana's. Probably the fastest two herbs which you can take are ginger (make a strong ginger tea) and Rauvolfia Serpentine, whereby effects can be noticed within 30 minutes. But other than that, most herbs take a few days to a week or two, to really demonstrate an effect.

So putting it all together means making slow progress and be willing to experiment. I know it feels little bit scary, when competed to a cookie cutter program, but then again cookie cutter programs don't work for most people, plus if a protocol is too difficult people will tend to drop out of it. Instead opt for a slow but steady rebalancing of your life, which means making some habit changes, learning how to relax, doing exercise and taking herbs. So this and you will be surprised at the changes which can take place over a 2 or 3 month period!

Finally as noted earlier in this book, high blood pressure levels vary from person to person. If you are borderline hypertensive, then chances are that you can undergo a complete cure, whereas as someone who has really high blood pressure levels, might be just looking at making a better overall balance. It's going to depend, so we can't guarantee a cure, but what can be guaranteed is a strong significant reduction in symptoms, over a period of months, if you explore with the various exercises, pranayama's herbs and lifestyles, as listed in this book!

And also the icing on the cake is that in the process of improving symptoms of high blood pressure you are actually curing your body and many health imbalances. As noted earlier, allopathic medicine sees high blood pressure as a disease and is basically concerned about chronic ill health, resulting out of the high blood pressure. Whereas from a complementary point of view, high blood pressure is the bodies way of coping with a more serious imbalance. So high blood pressure is simply a symptom of a bigger imbalance. Yes organic damage will occur from high blood pressure, over time, but also chronic ill health will result from the deficiencies present in our health, in the first place which have forced to body to develop high blood pressure!. So if you get a complete cure great, but even if you get a good reduction. in blood pressure level's, this suggests a good improvement in overall health and vitality levels... so keep it up!

Free Gifts

Bonus #1 – Grab Free Books!!!!!!!!

As a way of saying thank you for downloading this book I would like to give you two free books, which are available exclusively for my readers. The free book "Juicing for Health – 35 Juicing Recipes for Everyday Health Problems", is packed full of useful healthy juice recipes and Success Hacks - 31 Mind-Set Hacks to Increase Productivity and Career Success, is packed full of helpful mind hacks for developing a more dynamic and enjoyable lifestyle!

Thank You

I hope you have enjoyed this book and found it interesting. These herbs are very powerful and are a simple way to support you through the recovery process. But do remember they are a support so don't simply swap allopathic medications for herbs. Both allopathic and herbal formulations are simply there to assist you while you recover.

If you like this book please leave a review for it:

And for more interesting and helpful information, on every suspect of physical, mental, emotional and spiritual health, please visit my website:

healbodymindandspirit.com

Thanks once again for taking the time out to read this book.

Yours in health

Dermot Farrell

Appendix

1. http://www.who.int/gho/ncd/risk_factors/blood_pressure_prevalence_text/en/

2. http://www.worldometers.info/world-population/

3. http://wholehealthsource.blogspot.in/2012/02/by-2606-us-diet-will-be-100-percent.html

4. http://www.healthypeople.gov/2020/data/Chart/4947?category=926&by=Country_of_birth

5. http://www.heart.org/HEARTORG/Conditions/Cholesterol/PreventionTreatmentofHighCholesterol/Know-Your-Fats_UCM_305628_Article.jsp#.VnFYEUp97IU

6. http://www.heart.org/HEARTORG/Conditions/Cholesterol/PreventionTreatmentofHighCholesterol/Know-Your-Fats_UCM_305628_Article.jsp#.VnFYEUp97IU

7. http://www.cdc.gov/obesity/data/adult.html

8. http://articles.mercola.com/sites/articles/archive/2010/05/25/startling-research-findings-a-newly-discovered-cause-of-high-blood-pressure-and-obesity.aspx

9. http://www.americashealthrankings.org/FL/Hypertension

10. Effects of Cinnamon Consumption on Glycemic Status, Lipid Profile and Body Composition in Type 2 Diabetes Patients

Vafa, Mohammad Reza; Mohammadi, Farhad; Shidfar, Farzad; Mohammadhossein Salehi Sormaghi; Heidari, Iraj; et al. International Journal of Preventive Medicine 3.8 (Aug 2012): n/a.

11. Effect of garlic on blood pressure: A systematic review and meta-analysis
Karin RiedEmail author, Oliver R Frank, Nigel P Stocks, Peter Fakler and Thomas Sullivan
BMC Cardiovascular Disorders20088:13
DOI: 10.1186/1471-2261-8-13
© Ried et al. 2008
Received: 26 March 2008
Accepted: 16 June 2008
Published: 16 June 2008

12. J Agric Food Chem. 2010 Oct 13;58(19):10347-55. doi: 10.1021/jf101606s.
Cardiac contractile dysfunction and apoptosis in streptozotocin-induced diabetic rats are ameliorated by garlic oil supplementation.
Ou HC, Tzang BS, Chang MH, Liu CT, Liu HW, Lii CK, Bau DT, Chao PM, Kuo WW.

13. Saudi Med J. 2008 Sep;29(9):1280-4.
Investigation of the effect of ginger on the lipid levels. A double blind controlled clinical trial.
Alizadeh-Navaei R, Roozbeh F, Saravi M, Pouramir M, Jalali F, Moghadamnia AA.

14. J Cardiovasc Pharmacol. 2005 Jan;45(1):74-80.
Ginger lowers blood pressure through blockade of voltage-dependent calcium channels.
Ghavur MN, Gilani Ah

15. Verma S K, Jain Vartika, Katewa S S. Blood pressure lowering, fibrinolysis enhancing and antioxidant activities of Cardamom (Elettaria cardamomum). Indian Journal of Biochemistry & Biophysics. 2009 Dec; 46(6): 503-506.

www.ingramcontent.com/pod-product-compliance
Lightning Source LLC
Chambersburg PA
CBHW071419180526
45170CB00001B/156